Self-Care for Chronic Pain

Effective Strategies and Techniques for Managing Pain and Enhancing Well-Being

Jordan Taylor

INTRODUCTION

OVERVIEW OF CHRONIC PAIN

Chronic pain is a complex and multifaceted condition characterized by persistent discomfort that lasts beyond the usual course of acute illness or injury. Unlike acute pain, which serves as a warning system for potential harm and resolves as the underlying cause heals, chronic pain persists for months or even years, often without a clear or immediate cause.

Understanding Chronic Pain:
Chronic pain is typically defined as pain that lasts for longer than three to six months. It can arise from various sources, including:

- **Injuries or Trauma:** Pain from an injury or surgery that continues even after the physical damage has healed.

- **Medical Conditions**: Pain associated with conditions such as arthritis, fibromyalgia, or endometriosis.

- **Neuropathic Pain**: Pain resulting from nerve damage or dysfunction, often described as burning, tingling, or shooting sensations.

- **Unknown Origins:** Sometimes, the source of chronic pain may not be identifiable, making diagnosis and treatment more challenging.

The Biopsychosocial Model of Pain:
The experience of chronic pain is influenced by a combination of biological, psychological, and social factors, collectively referred to as the biopsychosocial model. This model recognizes that:

- Biological Factors: These include the physiological processes of pain, such as nerve damage or inflammation, as well as genetic predispositions that may affect pain sensitivity and response.

- Psychological Factors: Emotional states, such as depression and anxiety, can exacerbate the perception of pain. Cognitive processes, such as attention and coping strategies, also play a significant role.

- Social Factors: The impact of chronic pain on social relationships, work, and daily activities can affect an individual's overall well-being. Social support and the presence or absence of a support system can significantly influence pain management and recovery.
Impact on Daily Life:

Chronic pain can have a profound impact on various aspects of daily life, including:

- **Physical Functioning**: Persistent pain can limit mobility, reduce physical activity, and impair the ability to perform daily tasks. This can lead to physical deconditioning and further exacerbate pain symptoms.
- **Emotional Well-being:** Living with chronic pain can lead to emotional distress, including feelings of frustration, helplessness, and sadness. The constant struggle with pain can affect self-esteem and overall quality of life.
- **Social Relationships**: Chronic pain can strain relationships with family, friends, and colleagues. The limitations imposed by pain may lead to social isolation or misunderstandings from others who may not fully grasp the nature of the condition.
- **Work and Productivity**: Chronic pain can affect job performance and productivity. It may lead to absenteeism, reduced work capacity, and, in some cases, job loss. The financial implications of managing chronic pain, including medical expenses and potential loss of income, can add to the stress and burden.

Management and Treatment Approaches:
Managing chronic pain often requires a multifaceted approach, including:

- **Medical Interventions**: These may involve medications, physical therapy, and other medical treatments aimed at alleviating pain and addressing underlying conditions.

- **Self-Care Strategies:** Implementing self-care techniques such as exercise, stress management, and dietary adjustments can play a crucial role in managing chronic pain.

- **Psychological Support:** Counseling, cognitive-behavioral therapy (CBT), and other psychological interventions can help individuals cope with the emotional and mental aspects of chronic pain.

- **Alternative Therapies**: Complementary approaches, such as acupuncture, massage, and mindfulness practices, may provide additional relief and support.

IMPACT ON DAILY LIFE

Chronic pain is not just a physical sensation but a multifaceted experience that deeply affects nearly every aspect of an individual's daily life. The persistent nature of chronic pain can create a cascade of challenges that extend beyond the physical discomfort itself. Understanding these impacts is crucial for developing effective self-care strategies and support systems.

Physical Limitations and Functional Impairment:
Chronic pain often results in significant physical limitations and functional impairments that can alter a person's daily routine. Key aspects include:

- **Reduced Mobility:** Persistent pain can make it difficult to move freely and engage in activities that were once routine. Tasks such as walking, climbing stairs, or even standing for prolonged periods can become challenging. This reduction in mobility can lead to a more sedentary lifestyle, which may further contribute to physical deconditioning and exacerbate pain.
- **Impaired Physical Functioning**: Chronic pain can affect the ability to perform everyday tasks, including household chores, personal care, and recreational activities. Simple activities like cooking, cleaning, or gardening may become burdensome or impossible, impacting one's sense of independence and self-sufficiency.
- **Increased Fatigue:** Managing chronic pain can be physically exhausting. The constant strain of dealing with pain can lead to increased fatigue and a decreased ability to engage in physical activities. This fatigue can compound the physical challenges and diminish overall energy levels.

Emotional and Psychological Effects:
The emotional and psychological toll of chronic pain is profound, influencing mental health and overall well-being:

- **Emotional Distress:** Chronic pain is often associated with feelings of frustration, anger, and sadness. The relentless nature of the pain can lead to a sense of hopelessness and despair, impacting one's mood and emotional stability.
- **Anxiety and Depression**: Many individuals with chronic pain experience anxiety and depression as secondary conditions. The ongoing discomfort, coupled with uncertainty about the future, can contribute to heightened anxiety and depressive symptoms. This mental health burden can create a cycle of worsening pain and emotional distress.
- **Impact on Self-Esteem:** Persistent pain can affect self-esteem and body image. Individuals may feel inadequate or less capable due to their limitations, which can impact their self-worth and confidence. The inability to perform tasks or engage in activities they once enjoyed can lead to feelings of inadequacy and self-doubt.

Social and Relationship Challenges:
Chronic pain can strain relationships and social interactions, influencing both personal and professional connections:

- **Strain on Family and Social Relationships**: Chronic pain can place a significant burden on family members and friends. Caregivers may experience stress and fatigue, and the person with pain may feel guilty or burdensome. Misunderstandings or lack of empathy from others can further exacerbate feelings of isolation.
- **Social Isolation:** Due to physical limitations and emotional distress, individuals with chronic pain may withdraw from social activities and engagements. This withdrawal can lead to social isolation and reduced interaction with friends, family, and community, impacting overall social well-being.
- **Work and Career Impact:** Chronic pain can affect job performance and career advancement. Difficulties in maintaining consistent attendance, reduced productivity, and limitations in job duties can lead to job dissatisfaction, potential job loss, or career changes. The financial implications of these changes can add additional stress.

Financial and Practical Implications:

The economic burden of chronic pain can be substantial and multifaceted:

- **Medical Expenses:** Ongoing medical care, including doctor visits, medications, physical therapy, and alternative treatments, can result in significant financial costs. Insurance coverage may not fully address these expenses, leading to financial strain.

- **Loss of Income:** The inability to work or reduced work capacity can result in loss of income. This financial impact can affect the individual's quality of life and increase stress levels.

- **Cost of Assistive Devices and Modifications**: Individuals with chronic pain may require assistive devices or home modifications to accommodate their needs. These additional costs can further strain financial resources.

Overall Quality of Life:

The cumulative effect of these challenges can significantly diminish overall quality of life. Chronic pain can affect one's ability to enjoy life, pursue hobbies, and maintain a fulfilling and active lifestyle. The constant struggle with pain, combined with its wide-ranging impacts, can lead to a diminished sense of well-being and satisfaction.

Strategies for Coping and Management:

To address these impacts effectively, a comprehensive approach that includes self-care strategies, emotional support, and practical solutions is essential. This may involve:

- **Developing a Self-Care Routine**: Implementing a structured self-care routine that includes physical activity, relaxation techniques, and dietary adjustments can help manage symptoms and improve overall well-being.

- **Seeking Professional Support:** Engaging with healthcare professionals, including pain specialists, physical therapists, and mental health counselors, can provide valuable support and guidance.

- **Building a Support Network**: Connecting with support groups, friends, and family members can offer emotional and practical support, helping to alleviate feelings of isolation and stress.

PURPOSE AND SCOPE OF THIS BOOK

Purpose of the Book:
The primary purpose of "Self-Care for Chronic Pain: Effective Strategies and Techniques" is to provide a comprehensive and practical guide for individuals living with chronic pain. The book aims to empower readers with the knowledge, tools, and strategies necessary to

manage their condition more effectively and enhance their quality of life. It is designed to serve as both an educational resource and a practical handbook, addressing various aspects of chronic pain management from a holistic perspective.

Key Objectives:

1. **Educate on Chronic Pain**: To offer a thorough understanding of what chronic pain is, including its mechanisms, types, and impacts. By providing foundational knowledge, the book helps readers grasp the complexity of their condition and its implications for their daily lives.

2. **Promote Self-Care Strategies**: To introduce and elaborate on a range of self-care strategies that can help manage chronic pain. This includes physical therapies, mental health practices, dietary adjustments, and lifestyle changes that can contribute to better pain management and overall well-being.

3. **Support Emotional and Psychological Well-being:** To address the emotional and psychological aspects of chronic pain, including strategies for coping with anxiety, depression, and stress. The book aims to provide tools for managing the mental health challenges that often accompany chronic pain.

4. **Offer Practical Guidance**: To provide actionable advice and practical guidance on implementing self-care strategies. The book includes step-by-step instructions, tips, and techniques that readers can easily integrate into their daily routines.

5. **Encourage a Holistic Approach**: To emphasize the importance of a holistic approach to chronic pain management, considering the interplay of physical, emotional, and social factors. The book encourages readers to take a comprehensive approach to their care, incorporating various elements to address their unique needs.

Scope of the Book:

"Self-Care for Chronic Pain: Effective Strategies and Techniques" covers a wide range of topics essential for managing chronic pain effectively. The scope includes:

1. **Understanding Chronic Pain:**

   - An in-depth exploration of chronic pain, including its definitions, types, and underlying mechanisms.

   - Insights into how chronic pain affects the body and mind, including the biopsychosocial model that highlights the interaction of biological, psychological, and social factors.

2. **Self-Care Planning and Implementation:**
- Guidelines for developing a personalized self-care plan tailored to individual needs and pain levels.
- Strategies for setting realistic goals and incorporating self-care practices into daily life.

3. **Physical Therapy and Exercise:**
- Detailed information on physical therapy techniques and exercises that can help alleviate pain and improve physical functioning.
- Guidance on creating an effective exercise routine and working with physical therapists.

4. **Mindfulness and Stress Management:**
- Techniques for practicing mindfulness, managing stress, and incorporating relaxation exercises into daily life.
- Methods for using mindfulness and stress management to reduce the perception of pain and enhance emotional well-being.

5. **Nutrition and Diet:**
- The impact of diet on chronic pain, including recommendations for anti-inflammatory foods and dietary adjustments.

- Practical advice on creating a balanced diet plan to support overall health and manage pain.

6. **Pain Management Tools and Techniques:**
   - Overview of various tools and techniques for pain management, such as heat/cold therapy, massage, and acupuncture.
   - Guidance on using assistive devices and alternative therapies to complement traditional treatments.
7. Mental Health and Emotional Support:
   - Strategies for addressing the emotional and psychological challenges of living with chronic pain.
   - Information on seeking professional support, building a support network, and coping with emotional distress.
8. **Medications and Alternative Therapies:**
   - An overview of commonly used medications and alternative treatments for chronic pain.
   - Discussion on evaluating treatment options and working with healthcare providers to find effective solutions.
9. **Monitoring and Adjusting Your Plan:**
   - Methods for tracking pain levels and progress, assessing the effectiveness of self-care strategies, and making necessary adjustments.

- Tips for recognizing when additional help is needed and adapting your plan to achieve better outcomes.

10. Future Trends and Research:
   - Exploration of emerging treatments and research in chronic pain management.
   - Insights into potential future therapies and how to stay informed about advancements in the field.

Target Audience:
The book is intended for individuals living with chronic pain, their caregivers, and anyone seeking to understand and manage chronic pain more effectively. It is designed to be accessible to both newcomers to pain management and those who have been dealing with chronic pain for years. Healthcare professionals and support groups may also find the book useful as a resource for guiding patients and clients.

Structure and Approach:
The book is structured to provide a logical flow of information, starting with foundational knowledge and moving towards practical strategies and techniques. Each chapter is designed to build upon the previous one, ensuring that readers gain a comprehensive understanding of chronic pain and how to manage it effectively. The approach combines evidence-based

practices with practical advice, offering readers a well-rounded perspective on chronic pain management. By addressing the complexities of chronic pain through a multifaceted approach, this book aims to equip readers with the tools and knowledge necessary to take control of their condition and improve their overall quality of life.

HOW TO USE THIS GUIDE

"Self-Care for Chronic Pain: Effective Strategies and Techniques" is designed to be a practical and user-friendly resource for individuals dealing with chronic pain. To maximize the benefits of this guide, it's essential to understand how to navigate its contents effectively. This section provides a detailed explanation of how to use the book to its fullest potential.

1.4.1 Navigating the Book

Table of Contents:
Start by familiarizing yourself with the Table of Contents. This section provides an overview of the book's structure and helps you locate specific topics of interest quickly. The Table of Contents is organized into chapters and subchapters, each addressing a different aspect of chronic pain management.

Introduction:
Read the Introduction thoroughly. This section sets the stage for the rest of the book, explaining the purpose, scope, and objectives. It provides essential context and prepares you for the information and strategies presented in subsequent chapters.

Chapters and Subchapters:
Each chapter is divided into subchapters that focus on specific aspects of chronic pain management. The chapters are organized to build upon one another, starting with foundational knowledge and progressing to more advanced strategies. The subchapters within each chapter provide detailed information and practical advice on particular topics.

1.4.2 How to Approach Each Chapter

Read Sequentially or Selectively:
While the book is structured to be read from start to finish, you can also choose to focus on specific chapters that are most relevant to your needs. If you are new to chronic pain management, starting from the beginning and working through each chapter sequentially may provide a comprehensive understanding. If you have specific concerns or areas of interest, you can select chapters based on those needs.

Follow the Structure:

Each chapter follows a consistent structure to facilitate understanding and application. Typically, you will find the following components:

- **Introduction**: Provides an overview of the chapter's focus and sets the context.

- **Detailed Content:** Includes explanations, strategies, and techniques related to the chapter's topic. This section offers in-depth information and practical advice.

- **Practical Tips:** Highlights actionable tips and suggestions that can be implemented in daily life.

- **Case Studies and Examples**: Provides real-life examples or case studies to illustrate key points and offer practical insights.

- **Summary**: Summarizes the main points of the chapter and reinforces key takeaways.

Utilize Practical Exercises and Tools:

Many chapters include practical exercises, worksheets, or tools designed to help you apply the information to your personal situation. Engage with these exercises to tailor the strategies to your unique needs and track your progress.

Refer to Additional Resources:
Throughout the book, you may find references to additional resources, such as recommended readings, websites, or organizations. These resources can provide further information and support. Use them to deepen your understanding and enhance your chronic pain management efforts.

1.4.3 Implementing Self-Care Strategies
Develop a Personalized Plan:
Based on the information and strategies presented in the book, develop a personalized self-care plan. Consider your specific pain levels, lifestyle, and preferences when creating your plan. Incorporate the techniques and strategies that resonate with you and are feasible for your situation.

Set Realistic Goals:
Set achievable goals for implementing self-care strategies. Start with small, manageable changes and gradually build upon them. Setting realistic goals helps maintain motivation and allows you to track progress effectively.

Monitor and Evaluate:
Regularly monitor and evaluate the effectiveness of your self-care plan. Keep track of changes in your pain levels, physical functioning, and overall well-being. Make

adjustments as needed based on your observations and experiences.

Seek Professional Guidance:
While this guide provides valuable information and strategies, it is important to work with healthcare professionals to ensure a comprehensive approach to pain management. Consult with your doctor, physical therapist, or other healthcare providers for personalized advice and to address any medical concerns.

1.4.4 Building a Support Network
Connect with Support Groups:
Consider joining support groups or online communities for individuals with chronic pain. These groups can offer emotional support, practical advice, and a sense of camaraderie. Engaging with others who understand your experience can be beneficial for emotional well-being.

Involve Family and Friends:
Involve family and friends in your self-care efforts. Educate them about chronic pain and how they can support you. Open communication with loved ones can help reduce misunderstandings and create a supportive environment.

Professional Support:

Engage with mental health professionals, counselors, or therapists to address the emotional and psychological aspects of chronic pain. Professional support can provide valuable tools and strategies for managing stress, anxiety, and depression related to chronic pain.

1.4.5 Continuing Your Journey

Stay Informed:

Chronic pain management is an evolving field with ongoing research and new developments. Stay informed about the latest advancements and treatment options by following reputable sources, attending workshops, or reading current literature.

Adapt and Evolve:

Your needs and pain levels may change over time. Be prepared to adapt and evolve your self-care plan as necessary. Continuously evaluate your strategies and make adjustments based on your experiences and any new information you acquire.

Embrace a Holistic Approach:

Approach chronic pain management holistically by considering physical, emotional, and social aspects. Incorporate a variety of strategies to address different facets of your condition and enhance your overall quality of life.

CHAPTER 1

UNDERSTANDING CHRONIC PAIN

Chronic pain is a complex and multifaceted condition that extends beyond the typical duration of acute pain, persisting for weeks, months, or even years. It can have profound impacts on an individual's physical and emotional well-being. Understanding chronic pain involves recognizing its various definitions and types, which can help in developing effective management strategies. This chapter will delve into the definitions, classifications, and different types of chronic pain, providing a comprehensive overview of this challenging condition.

DEFINITION AND TYPES OF CHRONIC PAIN

Definition of Chronic Pain:
Chronic pain is defined as pain that persists beyond the usual course of acute illness or injury, typically lasting

longer than three to six months. Unlike acute pain, which is a direct response to tissue damage or injury and usually resolves with healing, chronic pain continues long after the initial cause has been treated or healed. Chronic pain can be persistent or intermittent, varying in intensity and severity over time.

This type of pain is often classified as either nociceptive or neuropathic, depending on its origin and underlying mechanisms. Understanding these definitions is crucial for effective diagnosis and management.

Nociceptive Pain:

Nociceptive pain results from damage or inflammation to body tissues and is typically described as sharp, aching, or throbbing. This type of pain serves as a protective mechanism, signaling that there is a potential or actual injury. It can be further divided into two categories:

- **Somatic Pain:** Originates from the skin, muscles, joints, or bones. It is usually localized and can be described as sharp, aching, or throbbing. Examples include pain from a cut, muscle strain, or joint injury.

- **Visceral Pain:** Arises from the internal organs such as the stomach, intestines, or bladder. It is often more diffuse and harder to localize. This type of pain can be described as deep, crampy, or pressure-like. Conditions such as irritable bowel syndrome (IBS) or chronic pelvic pain are examples of visceral pain.

Neuropathic Pain:
Neuropathic pain is caused by damage or dysfunction in the nervous system itself, rather than from tissue injury. This type of pain is often described as burning, tingling, or shooting and may be accompanied by numbness or hypersensitivity. Neuropathic pain can result from conditions such as:

- **Diabetic Neuropathy**: Nerve damage caused by diabetes, leading to pain and numbness, often in the hands and feet.
- **Postherpetic Neuralgia**: Pain that persists after a shingles outbreak, affecting the nerve pathways.
- **Fibromyalgia**: A condition characterized by widespread muscle pain and tenderness, thought to involve abnormal processing of pain signals in the brain and spinal cord.

Mixed Pain Syndromes:
Some chronic pain conditions involve a combination of nociceptive and neuropathic pain. For example:

Complex Regional Pain Syndrome (CRPS): A condition that usually follows an injury and involves both nociceptive and neuropathic pain. It is characterized by severe, continuous pain along with changes in skin color, temperature, and swelling in the affected limb.

- **Chronic Low Back Pain:** Often involves a mix of nociceptive pain from the muscles and ligaments and neuropathic pain from nerve involvement.

Acute vs. Chronic Pain:

Understanding the difference between acute and chronic pain is fundamental. Acute pain is a direct response to injury or illness and serves as a warning signal to protect the body. It usually resolves as the injury heals. In contrast, chronic pain persists long after the initial cause has been addressed and may continue despite apparent healing of the tissues.

Recurrent Pain:

Recurrent pain is characterized by episodes of pain that come and go, with periods of remission in between. This type of pain can occur in conditions like migraines or chronic headaches, where individuals experience episodic pain separated by pain-free intervals.

Impact of Chronic Pain:

Chronic pain can significantly impact an individual's quality of life, affecting physical function, emotional well-being, and daily activities. The persistence of pain can lead to psychological stress, changes in mood, and difficulties in maintaining social and occupational roles. It is crucial to address both the physical and emotional aspects of chronic pain for effective management.

PHYSIOLOGICAL MECHANISMS OF PAIN

Understanding the physiological mechanisms of pain is crucial for effective management and treatment of chronic pain. Pain is a complex experience that involves multiple systems within the body, including the nervous system, the immune system, and the brain. This section explores the intricate processes that contribute to the sensation and perception of pain, shedding light on how pain signals are generated, transmitted, and interpreted.

1.2.1 Pain Pathways

Nociceptors and Pain Receptors:

Pain begins with nociceptors, specialized sensory receptors that detect potentially harmful stimuli. These receptors are located throughout the body in tissues such as skin, muscles, joints, and organs. Nociceptors are sensitive to different types of stimuli, including mechanical (e.g., pressure or stretch), thermal (e.g., extreme temperatures), and chemical (e.g., inflammatory mediators).

When nociceptors are activated by noxious stimuli, they convert these stimuli into electrical signals through a process known as transduction. These electrical signals are then transmitted via peripheral nerves to the spinal cord and brain.

Transmission of Pain Signals:
The transmission of pain signals involves several steps:
- **Peripheral Nerves:** After transduction, pain signals travel along afferent nerve fibers, primarily A-delta fibers and C fibers. A-delta fibers are responsible for transmitting sharp, acute pain and have a myelinated structure that allows for faster signal conduction. C fibers, on the other hand, transmit dull, throbbing pain and are unmyelinated, resulting in slower signal conduction.
- **Spinal Cord Processing:** Pain signals reach the spinal cord, where they synapse with neurons in the dorsal horn. The spinal cord acts as a relay station, modulating and transmitting pain signals to the brain. This modulation can involve both excitatory and inhibitory mechanisms, affecting the intensity of the pain signal.
- **Ascending Pathways**: From the spinal cord, pain signals are transmitted to the brain via ascending pathways, including the spinothalamic tract. These

pathways carry the pain signals to various brain regions, including the thalamus, which acts as a relay center, and the somatosensory cortex, which processes the sensory aspects of pain.

- **Brain Processing:** The brain processes pain signals in several areas, including the thalamus, somatosensory cortex, limbic system, and prefrontal cortex. The somatosensory cortex interprets the location, intensity, and quality of pain, while the limbic system and prefrontal cortex are involved in the emotional and cognitive aspects of pain.

1.2.2 Pain Modulation

Endogenous Pain Modulation:
The body has its own pain modulation systems that can influence the perception of pain. These systems include:

- **Endogenous Opioids:** The body produces natural pain-relieving substances known as endogenous opioids, such as endorphins, enkephalins, and dynorphins. These molecules bind to opioid receptors in the nervous system, inhibiting pain transmission and providing analgesic effects.
- **Descending Pain Pathways**: The brain can modulate pain perception through descending pathways that project from the brainstem to the spinal cord. These pathways can either inhibit or facilitate pain signals. The release of neurotransmitters such as serotonin and

norepinephrine in the spinal cord can influence the pain experience.

- **Gate Control Theory:** This theory, proposed by Melzack and Wall, suggests that the spinal cord contains a "gate" mechanism that can modulate the flow of pain signals to the brain. Non-painful stimuli (e.g., touch or vibration) can activate large-diameter fibers that inhibit the transmission of pain signals carried by small-diameter fibers, effectively "closing the gate" to pain.

Chronic Pain and Sensitization:

In chronic pain conditions, the normal pain pathways can become altered, leading to heightened pain perception. Two key mechanisms involved in chronic pain include:

- **Central Sensitization:** This occurs when the central nervous system becomes hypersensitive to pain signals. Prolonged pain can lead to changes in spinal cord and brain function, resulting in increased responsiveness to pain stimuli and the development of pain in response to non-noxious stimuli.

- **Peripheral Sensitization:** This involves changes at the level of the nociceptors and peripheral nerves. Inflammatory mediators and ongoing tissue damage can lead to increased sensitivity of nociceptors, causing them to become more responsive to stimuli and contributing to chronic pain.

1.2.3 Neuroplasticity and Pain

Neuroplasticity:

Neuroplasticity refers to the ability of the nervous system to adapt and reorganize itself in response to experience and injury. In the context of chronic pain, neuroplastic changes can occur in both the peripheral and central nervous systems.

- **Peripheral Neuroplasticity:** Changes in peripheral nerve function, such as increased excitability or altered gene expression in nociceptors, can contribute to persistent pain.

- **Central Neuroplasticity:** The brain and spinal cord can undergo structural and functional changes in response to chronic pain. These changes may include alterations in brain connectivity, increased activation of pain-related brain regions, and rewiring of neural circuits involved in pain processing.

Impact of Neuroplasticity on Pain Perception:

Neuroplasticity can result in altered pain perception, where the brain may become more sensitive to pain signals or develop maladaptive pain responses. This can lead to persistent and often debilitating pain experiences, even in the absence of ongoing tissue damage.

1.2.4 Implications for Pain Management

Understanding the Physiological Mechanisms:

A thorough understanding of the physiological mechanisms of pain is essential for developing effective pain management strategies. By identifying the underlying processes that contribute to pain, healthcare providers can tailor treatments to address specific aspects of pain, such as reducing inflammation, modulating pain signals, or targeting neuroplastic changes.

Multidisciplinary Approach:
Effective pain management often requires a multidisciplinary approach that combines pharmacological treatments, physical therapy, psychological support, and lifestyle modifications. Addressing the physiological mechanisms of pain can help guide the selection of appropriate interventions and optimize treatment outcomes.

Future Research:
Ongoing research into the physiological mechanisms of pain aims to uncover new insights and develop innovative treatments. Advances in neuroscience, genetics, and pain physiology hold the potential to improve our understanding of chronic pain and lead to more targeted and effective therapies.

PSYCHOLOGICAL ASPECTS OF CHRONIC PAIN

Chronic pain is not only a physical experience but also deeply intertwined with psychological factors. The impact of chronic pain on mental health can be profound, influencing emotional well-being, cognitive processes, and overall quality of life. Understanding the psychological aspects of chronic pain is crucial for developing a holistic approach to pain management that addresses both physical and mental health. This section delves into various psychological factors that contribute to and are affected by chronic pain, including emotional responses, cognitive distortions, and behavioral changes.

Emotional Responses to Chronic Pain:

Chronic pain often triggers a range of emotional responses, which can significantly impact an individual's mental health. These emotional responses may include:

- **Depression**: Chronic pain is closely associated with an increased risk of depression. Persistent pain can lead to feelings of hopelessness, sadness, and a loss of interest in previously enjoyable activities. The constant struggle with pain can exacerbate depressive symptoms and lead to a vicious cycle where depression worsens the perception of pain.

- **Anxiety**: Individuals with chronic pain may experience heightened anxiety related to their condition. Worries about the future, the potential for worsening pain, and concerns about the impact of pain on daily life can contribute to anxiety. The fear of pain flare-ups and uncertainty about treatment outcomes can also amplify anxiety levels.

- **Anger and Frustration:** The experience of chronic pain can lead to feelings of anger and frustration. Individuals may feel frustrated with the limitations imposed by their pain, the lack of effective treatment options, or the impact of pain on their personal and professional lives. This anger can sometimes be directed toward oneself, healthcare providers, or loved ones.

Cognitive Distortions and Pain Perception:
Chronic pain can influence cognitive processes, leading to distorted thinking patterns that affect how pain is perceived and managed. Common cognitive distortions associated with chronic pain include:

- **Catastrophizing**: This cognitive distortion involves anticipating the worst possible outcomes and magnifying the negative aspects of pain. Individuals who catastrophize may believe that their pain will continue to worsen indefinitely, leading to increased distress and a sense of helplessness.

- **Overgeneralization:** Overgeneralization involves making broad, negative conclusions based on specific pain experiences. For example, an individual might generalize their pain from a particular activity to a belief that all activities will cause pain, leading to avoidance and reduced activity levels.

- **Selective Attention:** Chronic pain can lead to selective attention, where individuals focus primarily on pain-related stimuli and overlook other positive aspects of their lives. This heightened focus on pain can reinforce negative thoughts and exacerbate the experience of pain.

Behavioral Changes and Coping Strategies:
Chronic pain often results in behavioral changes that can impact an individual's overall well-being. Common behavioral changes associated with chronic pain include:

- **Activity Limitations:** Due to pain, individuals may reduce their level of physical activity, leading to decreased physical fitness and potential complications such as muscle atrophy or joint stiffness. Avoidance of activities that are perceived as painful can further contribute to physical deconditioning.

- **Social Withdrawal:** Chronic pain can lead to social withdrawal, where individuals isolate themselves from social interactions and activities. This withdrawal can result from embarrassment, fear of pain exacerbation, or the belief that others do not understand their condition.

- **Changes in Daily Routines:** Individuals with chronic pain may modify their daily routines to accommodate their pain. This can include changes in work schedules, household responsibilities, and leisure activities. While these modifications may be necessary, they can also contribute to a sense of loss and reduced quality of life.

Impact on Relationships:
The psychological aspects of chronic pain can strain relationships with family, friends, and colleagues. Key impacts include:
- **Communication Challenges:** Effective communication about pain can be challenging, as individuals may struggle to convey the intensity and impact of their pain to others. Misunderstandings and lack of empathy from loved ones can contribute to relationship strain.
- **Family Dynamics:** Chronic pain can affect family dynamics, with family members taking on caregiving roles or experiencing stress related to the individual's condition. The demands of caregiving and the emotional burden of supporting a loved one with chronic pain can impact family relationships and well-being.
- **Social Support:** Access to social support is crucial for managing chronic pain, but individuals may find it difficult to seek or receive adequate support. The quality and availability of social support can influence emotional resilience and overall coping strategies.

Psychological Assessment and Treatment:

Addressing the psychological aspects of chronic pain involves a comprehensive assessment and tailored treatment approaches. Key components include:

- **Psychological Assessment:** Conducting a thorough psychological assessment can help identify emotional and cognitive factors that contribute to the experience of pain. This assessment may involve interviews, self-report questionnaires, and behavioral observations.

- **Cognitive-Behavioral Therapy (CBT):** CBT is a common therapeutic approach for managing the psychological aspects of chronic pain. It focuses on identifying and challenging cognitive distortions, developing coping strategies, and improving emotional regulation. CBT can help individuals reframe their thoughts about pain and develop more adaptive behaviors.

- **Mindfulness and Relaxation Techniques:** Mindfulness-based approaches and relaxation techniques can help individuals manage the emotional and cognitive aspects of chronic pain. Practices such as mindfulness meditation, progressive muscle relaxation, and guided imagery can reduce stress, enhance relaxation, and improve overall well-being.

- **Support Groups:** Joining support groups for individuals with chronic pain can provide a valuable source of emotional support and practical advice. Sharing experiences with others who understand the challenges of chronic pain can foster a sense of connection and reduce feelings of isolation.

DIAGNOSING CHRONIC PAIN CONDITIONS

Diagnosing chronic pain conditions involves a multifaceted approach that includes a comprehensive assessment of the patient's medical history, physical examination, and diagnostic testing. Given the complex nature of chronic pain, accurately identifying the underlying causes and contributing factors is essential for developing effective treatment strategies. This section explores the various methods and processes involved in diagnosing chronic pain, including the roles of clinical evaluation, diagnostic imaging, laboratory tests, and interdisciplinary collaboration.

Clinical Evaluation:
Medical History:
A detailed medical history is crucial in diagnosing chronic pain conditions. This history includes information about:
- Pain Onset and Duration: Understanding when the pain began, its progression, and how long it has persisted

helps in identifying potential causes and determining whether the pain is acute or chronic.

- Pain Characteristics: Describing the nature of the pain, such as its location, intensity, quality (e.g., sharp, dull, throbbing), and duration, provides insights into the possible underlying conditions. Additionally, noting factors that exacerbate or relieve the pain can aid in diagnosis.

- Previous Medical Conditions: Reviewing the patient's past medical conditions, surgeries, injuries, or illnesses can reveal connections between previous events and the current pain condition.

- Family History: Assessing family history of chronic pain conditions or other relevant medical conditions can help identify genetic or hereditary factors that might contribute to the pain.

- Psychosocial Factors: Understanding the patient's psychological and social background, including stress levels, mental health issues, and lifestyle factors, is essential for a comprehensive diagnosis.

Physical Examination:
A thorough physical examination involves:
- **Inspection and Palpation**: Visual inspection and palpation of the affected areas can help identify signs of inflammation, swelling, tenderness, or abnormalities in the musculoskeletal system.

- **Range of Motion Testing**: Assessing the range of motion in the affected areas can help determine if pain is related to joint or muscle issues. Limited range of motion may indicate stiffness, joint dysfunction, or muscular problems.

- **Neurological Examination**: Evaluating neurological function, including reflexes, sensation, and motor function, helps identify potential nerve involvement or neuropathic pain.

Diagnostic Imaging:
X-rays:
X-rays are commonly used to visualize bone structures and detect abnormalities such as fractures, dislocations, and degenerative changes. They are particularly useful for diagnosing conditions like osteoarthritis and spinal issues.

Magnetic Resonance Imaging (MRI):
MRI provides detailed images of soft tissues, including muscles, ligaments, and intervertebral discs. It is valuable for diagnosing conditions such as herniated discs, spinal stenosis, and soft tissue injuries. MRI can also help evaluate the extent of damage and guide treatment planning.

Computed Tomography (CT) Scans:

CT scans offer detailed cross-sectional images of the body and are useful for diagnosing bone and joint abnormalities, as well as detecting tumors or other structural issues. They are often used when MRI is not available or suitable for the patient.

Ultrasound:
Ultrasound imaging uses sound waves to visualize soft tissues and assess conditions such as tendinitis, bursitis, and muscle tears. It is also used for guided injections and to monitor changes in soft tissue structures.

Diagnostic Laboratory Tests:
Blood Tests:
Blood tests can help identify systemic conditions or markers of inflammation that may contribute to chronic pain. Tests may include:
- **Complete Blood Count (CBC)**: Evaluates overall health and detects signs of infection, anemia, or other hematological issues.
- **Erythrocyte Sedimentation Rate (ESR) and C-Reactive Protein (CRP)**: Measure levels of inflammation in the body. Elevated levels may indicate inflammatory or autoimmune conditions.
- **Rheumatoid Factor (RF) and Antinuclear Antibody (ANA) Tests**: Assess for autoimmune disorders such as

rheumatoid arthritis or lupus, which can cause chronic pain.

Urine Tests:

Urine tests may be used to assess kidney function, detect metabolic disorders, or identify signs of infection. These tests can provide additional information about underlying conditions that may contribute to chronic pain.

Specialized Tests:

- **Electromyography (EMG) and Nerve Conduction Studies**: Evaluate electrical activity in muscles and nerves, helping to diagnose neuropathies and neuromuscular disorders.

- **Bone Scintigraphy (Bone Scan):** Uses radioactive tracers to detect bone abnormalities, such as infections, tumors, or fractures not visible on standard X-rays.

Interdisciplinary Approach:

Referral to Specialists:

In complex cases, referral to specialists may be necessary for a comprehensive evaluation. Specialists may include:

- **Rheumatologists:** Experts in autoimmune and inflammatory conditions.

- **Orthopedic Surgeons:** Specialists in musculoskeletal disorders and injuries.

- **Neurologists:** Experts in neurological conditions affecting pain perception.

- Pain Management Specialists: Focus on diagnosing and treating various pain conditions using multimodal approaches.

Multidisciplinary Evaluation:
A multidisciplinary approach involves collaboration among healthcare providers, including primary care physicians, pain specialists, physical therapists, psychologists, and occupational therapists. This approach ensures a comprehensive assessment of both physical and psychological factors contributing to chronic pain.

Diagnostic Challenges:
Diagnosing chronic pain can be challenging due to:
- Subjectivity: Pain is a subjective experience, making it difficult to measure and quantify. Patient self-reports and assessments are crucial for understanding the impact of pain.
- Overlap of Symptoms: Many chronic pain conditions share similar symptoms, making differential diagnosis challenging. Careful evaluation and exclusion of other conditions are necessary to arrive at an accurate diagnosis.
- Lack of Definitive Tests: Unlike some medical conditions, chronic pain often lacks definitive diagnostic tests. Diagnosis is based on a combination of clinical evaluation, imaging, and laboratory tests.

CHAPTER 2

MANAGING CHRONIC PAIN

Effective management of chronic pain often requires a multifaceted approach that includes pharmacological treatments, physical therapies, psychological interventions, and lifestyle modifications. This chapter explores various strategies for managing chronic pain, with a particular focus on pharmacological treatments, which play a critical role in alleviating pain and improving quality of life. The section will provide an in-depth look at different classes of medications, their mechanisms of action, and considerations for their use.

PHARMACOLOGICAL TREATMENTS

Pharmacological treatments are a cornerstone in managing chronic pain, offering relief through various types of medications. These treatments aim to alleviate pain, improve function, and enhance overall quality of life. The choice of medication depends on the type, severity, and underlying cause of the pain, as well as individual patient factors. This section provides a comprehensive overview of the primary classes of medications used in chronic pain management, including their mechanisms of action, potential benefits, and possible side effects.

Non-Opioid Analgesics:

Non-opioid analgesics are commonly used to manage mild to moderate pain and are often the first line of treatment. These medications work by interfering with the body's pain signaling pathways and can be effective for various types of pain, including musculoskeletal pain and headaches.

- **Acetaminophen:** Acetaminophen is a widely used analgesic that works primarily in the central nervous system to reduce pain and fever. It is effective for mild to moderate pain, such as headaches, muscle aches, and osteoarthritis. While generally well-tolerated, overuse of acetaminophen can lead to liver damage. It is important to adhere to recommended dosing guidelines to avoid potential toxicity.

- **Non-Steroidal Anti-Inflammatory Drugs (NSAIDs):** NSAIDs, including ibuprofen, naproxen, and aspirin, are used to manage pain and inflammation. They work by inhibiting the production of prostaglandins, which are chemicals involved in inflammation and pain. NSAIDs are effective for conditions such as arthritis, back pain, and menstrual cramps. Potential side effects include gastrointestinal irritation, ulcers, and increased risk of cardiovascular events, especially with long-term use.

Opioids:

Opioids are powerful analgesics used for managing severe pain, particularly when non-opioid treatments are insufficient. They act on opioid receptors in the central nervous system to block pain signals and produce a sense of euphoria. Opioids can be highly effective but carry risks of dependence, addiction, and overdose.

- **Common Opioids:** Examples include morphine, oxycodone, hydrocodone, and fentanyl. These medications vary in potency and duration of action. They are typically used for short-term management of acute pain or for chronic pain when other options have failed.

- **Mechanism of Action:** Opioids bind to specific receptors in the brain and spinal cord, modulating the perception of pain. While effective at reducing pain, their use must be carefully managed to mitigate risks of side effects and long-term complications.

- **Side Effects and Risks:** Common side effects include constipation, nausea, drowsiness, and dizziness. Long-term use can lead to tolerance, physical dependence, and addiction. Strategies for managing opioid therapy include using the lowest effective dose for the shortest duration necessary and considering opioid-sparing approaches.

Adjuvant Medications:

Adjuvant medications are used alongside primary analgesics to enhance pain relief or address specific aspects of pain. These medications can be particularly useful for neuropathic pain or pain associated with certain conditions.

- **Antidepressants**: Certain antidepressants, such as tricyclic antidepressants (e.g., amitriptyline) and selective serotonin-norepinephrine reuptake inhibitors (e.g., duloxetine), can be effective in managing chronic pain, particularly neuropathic pain. They work by altering neurotransmitter levels in the brain, which can influence pain perception and mood.

- **Anticonvulsants**: Medications like gabapentin and pregabalin are used to manage neuropathic pain. They work by modulating nerve activity and reducing the abnormal electrical signals that contribute to pain.

- **Topical Analgesics:** Topical treatments, such as lidocaine patches or capsaicin creams, can be applied directly to the skin over painful areas. They provide localized pain relief with minimal systemic effects. Topical analgesics are often used for conditions like osteoarthritis or localized neuropathic pain.

Opioid Alternatives and Combination Therapies:

Given the risks associated with opioid use, there is growing interest in opioid alternatives and combination therapies that aim to provide effective pain relief while minimizing the risk of dependence and other adverse effects.

- **Combination Medications:** Combining medications with different mechanisms of action can enhance pain relief and reduce the need for high doses of any single medication. For example, combining an opioid with acetaminophen or an NSAID can provide better pain control than either medication alone.

- **Non-Pharmacological Adjuncts:** Integrating non-pharmacological treatments, such as physical therapy, cognitive-behavioral therapy, and alternative therapies (e.g., acupuncture), can improve overall pain management and reduce reliance on medications.

Monitoring and Adjusting Treatment:

Effective management of chronic pain requires ongoing monitoring and adjustment of treatment plans. Regular follow-up appointments with healthcare providers allow for:

- **Assessment of Treatment Efficacy**: Evaluating the effectiveness of medications and their impact on pain levels, functional status, and quality of life.

- **Management of Side Effects:** Identifying and addressing any side effects or adverse reactions to medications.

- **Adjusting Dosages:** Modifying medication dosages or switching to different medications based on the patient's response and evolving needs.

- **Patient Education:** Providing patients with information on medication use, potential side effects, and strategies for managing chronic pain.

SETTING REALISTIC GOALS

Setting realistic goals is a fundamental aspect of managing chronic pain. Effective goal-setting helps patients and healthcare providers create actionable plans that enhance pain management, improve quality of life, and promote overall well-being. Realistic goals are tailored to individual needs, capabilities, and circumstances, and they consider the complexities of chronic pain and its impact on daily life. This section explores the principles of setting realistic goals, strategies for developing and achieving them, and the importance of goal-setting in chronic pain management.

Principles of Setting Realistic Goals:
Individualization:
Realistic goals must be tailored to each patient's unique situation. Chronic pain affects individuals differently based on its type, severity, duration, and underlying causes. Therefore, goals should be personalized to reflect the patient's:

- **Pain Level and Functionality:** Goals should consider the patient's current level of pain and functional abilities. For instance, a patient with severe pain may have different goals compared to someone with moderate pain.

- **Physical and Emotional State:** Individual goals should account for the patient's overall physical health, emotional well-being, and psychological resilience. These factors influence the patient's ability to engage in and achieve goals.

- **Daily Activities and Lifestyle**: Goals should align with the patient's daily routines, work responsibilities, and lifestyle preferences. This alignment helps ensure that goals are practical and achievable within the patient's existing framework.

Incremental Progress:

Setting incremental goals helps in making gradual progress toward managing chronic pain. Smaller, manageable goals allow patients to:

- **Experience Achievable Success**: Breaking down larger goals into smaller steps provides a sense of accomplishment and motivation. Achieving these smaller goals reinforces positive behavior and encourages continued effort.

- **Adjust as Needed:** Incremental goals allow for flexibility and adjustments based on the patient's progress and changing needs. This adaptability helps in maintaining a realistic and effective approach to pain management.

Measurability:

Goals should be specific and measurable to track progress and assess effectiveness. Measurable goals include:

- **Quantifiable Metrics:** Setting goals with specific, quantifiable targets (e.g., reducing pain levels by a certain percentage, increasing mobility range) allows for objective evaluation of progress.

- **Clear Benchmarks:** Establishing clear benchmarks helps in monitoring achievements and identifying areas needing improvement. For example, a benchmark could be achieving a certain number of pain-free days per week.

Achievability:

Goals must be attainable and realistic given the patient's current condition and resources. To ensure achievability:

- **Consider Limitations:** Goals should reflect the patient's physical, emotional, and social limitations. Setting goals that are too ambitious or unrealistic can lead to frustration and discouragement.

- **Resource Availability:** Goals should be aligned with available resources, such as medical treatments, support systems, and financial means. Ensuring that goals are feasible with the resources at hand enhances the likelihood of success.

Relevance:
Goals should be relevant to the patient's overall health and well-being. Relevant goals focus on:
- **Priorities and Values:** Goals should align with what is most important to the patient, such as improving quality of life, maintaining independence, or participating in meaningful activities.
- **Long-Term Objectives:** Goals should support the patient's long-term objectives and aspirations. For example, a goal of improving physical function may align with the long-term objective of returning to a preferred hobby or activity.

Strategies for Developing and Achieving Goals:

Collaborative Goal Setting:
Collaborative goal setting involves working closely with healthcare providers, patients, and their families to establish goals. This collaboration ensures:
- **Patient Involvement:** Patients should be actively involved in setting their own goals to ensure they are meaningful and motivating. Engaging patients in the process fosters ownership and commitment to achieving the goals.

- **Healthcare Provider Input:** Healthcare providers offer expertise and guidance in setting realistic and achievable goals based on their assessment of the patient's condition and needs.

Action Plans:
Developing detailed action plans outlines the steps required to achieve each goal. Action plans should include:
- **Specific Actions:** Clearly defined actions that need to be taken to reach the goal. For example, if the goal is to improve physical activity, specific actions might include participating in physical therapy sessions or engaging in regular exercise routines.
- **Timeline**: A timeline for achieving each goal and its associated actions. Setting deadlines helps in organizing efforts and maintaining focus on progress.
- **Support and Resources:** Identifying the support systems and resources needed to achieve the goals. This may include accessing medical treatments, therapeutic interventions, or social support networks.

Monitoring and Evaluation:
Regular monitoring and evaluation are crucial for assessing progress and making necessary adjustments. This process involves:
- **Tracking Progress**: Keeping track of progress through regular assessments and evaluations. This may include

monitoring pain levels, functional improvements, or adherence to action plans.

- **Adjusting Goals:** Making adjustments to goals as needed based on the patient's progress, challenges, or changing circumstances. Flexibility ensures that goals remain relevant and achievable.

- **Celebrating Success:** Recognizing and celebrating successes, both small and large, reinforces positive behavior and motivates continued effort. Celebrations can enhance patient morale and encourage persistence.

Challenges and Solutions:

Overcoming Obstacles:

Patients may encounter obstacles in achieving their goals, such as:

- **Fluctuations in Pain Levels**: Pain levels may vary, impacting the ability to achieve goals. Developing strategies to manage pain fluctuations and adjusting goals accordingly can help overcome this challenge.

- **Limited Resources:** Resource limitations, such as financial constraints or lack of access to medical treatments, may affect goal achievement. Exploring alternative resources and support options can address this challenge.

Maintaining Motivation:

Maintaining motivation can be challenging, especially when progress is slow or setbacks occur. Strategies to maintain motivation include:

- **Setting Realistic Expectations:** Understanding that progress may be gradual and setting realistic expectations helps manage frustration and sustain motivation.

- **Seeking Support:** Engaging with support groups, counseling, or therapy can provide encouragement and motivation. Sharing experiences and challenges with others can offer additional support and perspective.

INTEGRATING SELF-CARE INTO DAILY ROUTINE

Integrating self-care into a daily routine is a crucial aspect of managing chronic pain. Self-care encompasses a variety of practices and strategies that individuals can adopt to enhance their physical, emotional, and mental well-being. Incorporating self-care into daily routines helps individuals manage their pain more effectively, improve overall quality of life, and foster a sense of empowerment and control over their condition. This section explores the principles of self-care, practical strategies for integration, and the benefits of adopting a self-care routine.

Principles of Self-Care:
Holistic Approach:
Self-care should address all aspects of an individual's well-being, including physical, emotional, and mental health. A holistic approach involves:
- Physical Health: Incorporating practices that support physical health, such as exercise, proper nutrition, and adequate sleep. Physical self-care helps in managing pain, improving strength and flexibility, and maintaining overall health.
- Emotional and Mental Health: Addressing emotional and mental well-being through activities that reduce stress, enhance mood, and promote mental resilience. This can include mindfulness practices, relaxation techniques, and engaging in enjoyable activities.
- Social and Environmental Factors: Considering the impact of social interactions and environmental conditions on well-being. Positive social connections and a supportive environment contribute to overall health and effective pain management.

Consistency:
Consistency in self-care practices is essential for achieving long-term benefits. Regularly incorporating self-care activities into daily routines helps in:
- Building Habits: Establishing a routine of self-care activities helps in creating lasting habits that become an integral part of daily life. Consistent practice enhances

the effectiveness of self-care and supports ongoing pain management.

- Managing Expectations: Setting realistic expectations and understanding that self-care is a continuous process. Consistency in practice helps in managing chronic pain more effectively and improving overall well-being.

Personalization:

Self-care practices should be personalized to meet individual needs and preferences. Personalization involves:

- Identifying Preferences: Choosing self-care activities that align with personal preferences and interests. Engaging in activities that are enjoyable and fulfilling increases adherence to self-care routines.

- Adapting to Needs: Adjusting self-care practices based on individual needs, pain levels, and daily circumstances. Flexibility in adapting self-care routines ensures that they remain effective and relevant.

Practical Strategies for Integration:

Creating a Self-Care Plan:

Developing a structured self-care plan helps in systematically incorporating self-care practices into daily routines. A self-care plan should include:

- Identifying Self-Care Activities: Listing activities that support physical, emotional, and mental well-being. Examples include exercise, meditation, hobbies, and social interactions.
- Setting Goals: Establishing specific, achievable goals for self-care activities. Goals can include daily, weekly, or monthly targets for engaging in self-care practices.
- Scheduling Time: Allocating dedicated time for self-care activities within the daily schedule. Incorporating self-care into regular routines ensures that it becomes a consistent practice.

Physical Self-Care:
Exercise and Physical Activity:
Regular exercise and physical activity are crucial for managing chronic pain and maintaining overall health. Strategies for integrating exercise into a daily routine include:
- Choosing Activities: Selecting exercises that are suitable for individual capabilities and preferences. Low-impact activities, such as walking, swimming, or gentle stretching, can be effective for managing pain and improving physical function.
- Establishing a Routine: Creating a regular exercise routine that includes daily or weekly sessions. Consistency in physical activity helps in building strength, improving flexibility, and reducing pain.

- Monitoring Progress: Tracking progress and adjusting exercise routines based on changes in pain levels and physical capabilities. Setting achievable milestones and celebrating successes can enhance motivation.

Nutrition and Hydration:
A balanced diet and proper hydration support overall health and can impact pain management. Key considerations include:
- Balanced Diet: Incorporating a variety of nutrient-rich foods, such as fruits, vegetables, whole grains, lean proteins, and healthy fats. A balanced diet supports energy levels, immune function, and overall well-being.
- Hydration: Ensuring adequate fluid intake throughout the day. Proper hydration supports bodily functions and can help in reducing the risk of dehydration-related symptoms.
- Avoiding Triggers: Identifying and avoiding dietary triggers that may exacerbate pain or inflammation. Consulting with a healthcare provider or nutritionist can help in developing a diet plan tailored to individual needs.

Sleep and Rest:
Adequate sleep and rest are essential for managing chronic pain and supporting overall health. Strategies for improving sleep quality include:

- **Establishing a Sleep Routine:** Creating a consistent sleep schedule with regular bedtimes and wake times. Consistent sleep patterns support better sleep quality and overall health.
- **Creating a Restful Environment:** Ensuring a comfortable and conducive sleep environment by controlling factors such as noise, light, and temperature. A restful environment promotes better sleep quality.
- **Incorporating Rest Periods:** Allowing for regular rest periods throughout the day to manage fatigue and prevent overexertion. Incorporating short breaks and relaxation techniques can help in maintaining energy levels.

Emotional and Mental Self-Care:
Mindfulness and Relaxation Techniques:
Mindfulness and relaxation techniques help in managing stress and enhancing emotional well-being. Strategies include:
- Mindfulness Meditation: Practicing mindfulness meditation to increase awareness of the present moment and reduce stress. Techniques such as deep breathing, body scans, and guided imagery can be effective.
- Relaxation Exercises: Engaging in relaxation exercises, such as progressive muscle relaxation or deep breathing exercises. These techniques help in reducing tension and promoting a sense of calm.

- Journaling: Keeping a journal to track emotions, thoughts, and experiences. Journaling can provide insight into emotional patterns and help in managing stress and anxiety.

Engaging in Enjoyable Activities:
Participating in activities that bring joy and fulfillment contributes to emotional well-being. Strategies include:
- Hobbies and Interests: Engaging in hobbies and activities that are enjoyable and meaningful. Pursuing personal interests provides a sense of accomplishment and enhances overall mood.
- Social Connections: Maintaining positive social connections and engaging in social activities. Building and nurturing relationships provide support, encouragement, and a sense of belonging.

Social Support and Connections:
Building a Support Network:
Developing a strong support network is essential for managing chronic pain and maintaining emotional well-being. Strategies include:
- Connecting with Others: Building relationships with family, friends, and support groups. Social connections provide emotional support, encouragement, and practical assistance.
- Seeking Professional Support: Engaging with healthcare providers, counselors, or therapists for

additional support. Professional support can offer guidance, coping strategies, and therapeutic interventions.

Maintaining a Supportive Environment:

Creating a supportive environment involves:

- Creating a Positive Home Environment: Ensuring that the home environment is conducive to relaxation and well-being. This may include organizing living spaces, reducing stressors, and promoting comfort.

- Accessing Community Resources: Utilizing community resources, such as support groups, educational programs, and wellness initiatives. Community resources provide additional support and opportunities for connection.

EVALUATING AND ADJUSTING YOUR PLAN

Evaluating and adjusting your chronic pain management plan is a crucial aspect of ensuring its effectiveness and optimizing outcomes. Chronic pain is a dynamic condition, and the strategies that work initially may require modification over time due to changes in symptoms, lifestyle, or overall health. This section explores the principles of evaluation and adjustment, strategies for assessing the effectiveness of a management plan, and methods for making necessary adjustments to enhance pain control and improve quality of life.

Principles of Evaluation and Adjustment:
Continuous Assessment:
Regular assessment of the pain management plan is essential for identifying what is working and what may need modification. Continuous assessment involves:
- Ongoing Monitoring: Keeping track of pain levels, functional abilities, and overall well-being on a regular basis. This can include daily or weekly monitoring of symptoms, treatment responses, and the impact of self-care practices.
- Feedback Collection: Gathering feedback from the patient regarding their experiences with the pain management plan. This feedback provides valuable insights into the effectiveness of various strategies and helps in identifying areas for improvement.

Flexibility:
A flexible approach to pain management allows for adjustments based on changing needs and circumstances. Flexibility involves:
- Adaptability: Being open to modifying the plan as needed based on changes in pain levels, physical capabilities, or personal circumstances. Flexibility ensures that the plan remains relevant and effective over time.

- - Response to Feedback: Incorporating feedback from patients and healthcare providers to make necessary adjustments. Responsive adjustments help in addressing new challenges and enhancing the overall effectiveness of the plan.

Collaborative Approach:

Evaluating and adjusting the pain management plan should involve collaboration between patients and healthcare providers. A collaborative approach ensures:

- Patient Involvement: Actively involving patients in the evaluation process to understand their experiences, preferences, and challenges. Patient input is crucial for making informed decisions about adjustments to the plan.

- Healthcare Provider Guidance: Seeking guidance and recommendations from healthcare providers based on their expertise and assessment of the patient's condition. Healthcare providers offer valuable insights into potential adjustments and alternative strategies.

Strategies for Evaluating the Effectiveness of the Plan:

Regular Check-Ins:

Scheduled check-ins with healthcare providers or pain management specialists help in assessing the effectiveness of the plan. Key components of check-ins include:

- Review of Goals: Evaluating progress toward established goals and determining whether they are being met. Reviewing goals helps in assessing whether the current strategies are effective or need adjustment.

- Symptom Tracking: Analyzing changes in pain levels, symptom frequency, and severity. Tracking symptoms helps in understanding the impact of the pain management plan and identifying areas needing modification.

- Functional Assessment: Assessing changes in physical function, mobility, and daily activities. Improvements or declines in functional abilities provide insight into the effectiveness of the plan.

Feedback Mechanisms:

Incorporating feedback mechanisms allows for a comprehensive evaluation of the plan's effectiveness. Feedback mechanisms include:

- Patient Surveys: Using surveys or questionnaires to gather feedback from patients about their experiences with the pain management plan. Surveys can assess various aspects, including pain relief, satisfaction with treatments, and overall quality of life.

- Self-Assessment Tools: Utilizing self-assessment tools to evaluate the impact of pain on daily life and well-being. Tools such as pain scales, activity logs, and mood assessments provide valuable information for evaluation.

Assessing Outcomes:
Evaluating the outcomes of the pain management plan involves analyzing both short-term and long-term results. Key outcomes to assess include:
- Pain Reduction: Measuring the extent of pain reduction achieved through the plan. This can include changes in pain intensity, frequency, and duration.
- Improved Functionality: Assessing improvements in physical function, mobility, and ability to perform daily activities. Functional improvements indicate the effectiveness of the plan in enhancing quality of life.
- Emotional Well-Being: Evaluating changes in emotional and mental well-being, such as mood, stress levels, and overall psychological health. Positive changes in emotional well-being reflect the impact of the plan on overall quality of life.

Methods for Adjusting the Plan:
Modifying Treatments:
Adjustments to treatments may be necessary based on the evaluation results. Methods for modifying treatments include:
- Changing Medications: Adjusting medication dosages, switching medications, or exploring alternative treatments based on effectiveness and side effects.

Consultation with a healthcare provider is essential for making safe and informed changes.

- Enhancing Therapies: Incorporating additional therapeutic interventions, such as physical therapy, occupational therapy, or complementary therapies. Enhancing therapies can address specific needs and improve overall pain management.

- Adjusting Pain Management Techniques: Modifying pain management techniques, such as relaxation exercises, mindfulness practices, or lifestyle changes. Adjustments should be based on the effectiveness and feasibility of the techniques.

Revising Goals:

Revising goals helps in aligning the pain management plan with current needs and priorities. Methods for revising goals include:

- Setting New Goals: Establishing new goals based on changes in pain levels, functional abilities, or personal circumstances. New goals should be realistic and achievable, reflecting the patient's current situation.

- Adjusting Existing Goals: Modifying existing goals to better align with progress and evolving needs. Adjustments should consider the patient's achievements, challenges, and changing priorities.

Updating Self-Care Practices:

Adjusting self-care practices ensures that they remain effective and relevant. Methods for updating self-care practices include:

- Incorporating New Strategies: Introducing new self-care strategies or modifying existing ones based on effectiveness and patient feedback. Exploring new techniques or activities can enhance overall self-care.

- Adapting to Changes: Adapting self-care practices based on changes in pain levels, physical abilities, or daily routines. Flexibility in self-care practices helps in maintaining effectiveness and addressing new challenges.

Addressing Challenges:

Identifying and addressing challenges that may impact the effectiveness of the plan is crucial. Methods for addressing challenges include:

- Problem-Solving: Identifying barriers or obstacles to achieving goals and developing strategies to overcome them. Problem-solving involves finding solutions to challenges such as medication side effects, lack of support, or logistical issues.

- Seeking Support: Engaging with healthcare providers, support groups, or counseling services to address challenges and gain additional guidance. Support networks provide valuable resources and assistance in managing difficulties.

CHAPTER 3

PHYSICAL THERAPY AND EXERCISE

BENEFITS OF PHYSICAL ACTIVITY

Physical activity plays a crucial role in the management of chronic pain and overall well-being. Engaging in regular exercise offers numerous benefits, from improving physical function to enhancing emotional health. This section delves into the multifaceted advantages of physical activity, explores how exercise can positively impact chronic pain conditions, and provides insights into integrating physical activity into a comprehensive pain management plan.

Improvement in Physical Function:
Enhancing Mobility and Flexibility:
Regular physical activity helps in improving mobility and flexibility, which are often compromised in individuals with chronic pain. Benefits include:
- Increased Range of Motion: Exercises that focus on stretching and flexibility help to maintain and improve the range of motion in affected joints and muscles. This can alleviate stiffness and enhance overall movement.
- Improved Joint Health: Weight-bearing exercises and stretching contribute to healthier joints by maintaining

cartilage integrity and promoting fluid movement. This helps in reducing joint pain and preventing further deterioration.

Strength Building:
Strengthening exercises, such as resistance training, play a significant role in managing chronic pain by:
- Muscle Support: Strengthening muscles around affected areas provides better support to joints and reduces strain. Stronger muscles help in stabilizing the body and reducing the risk of injury.
- Enhanced Endurance: Improved muscle strength leads to better endurance and stamina, enabling individuals to engage in daily activities with less fatigue and discomfort.

Pain Reduction:
Endorphin Release:
Physical activity stimulates the release of endorphins, which are natural painkillers produced by the body. The effects include:
- Pain Relief: Endorphins interact with the brain's pain receptors to diminish the perception of pain. This natural analgesic effect helps in reducing pain levels and enhancing overall comfort.
- Mood Enhancement: Endorphins also contribute to improved mood and emotional well-being, which can positively impact the perception of pain and stress levels.

Reduced Muscle Tension:
Exercise helps in relieving muscle tension and stiffness, which are common in chronic pain conditions. Benefits include:
- Relaxation: Physical activity promotes relaxation of tense muscles through increased blood flow and reduced muscle tightness. This can alleviate discomfort and improve overall muscle function.
- Reduced Spasms: Engaging in regular exercise can help prevent or reduce muscle spasms and cramping, which are often associated with chronic pain conditions.

Enhanced Overall Well-Being:
Improved Sleep Quality:
Regular physical activity contributes to better sleep quality, which is crucial for managing chronic pain. Benefits include:
- Regulated Sleep Patterns: Exercise helps in establishing consistent sleep patterns by promoting the release of sleep-regulating hormones. This leads to improved sleep duration and quality.
- Reduced Sleep Disturbances: Engaging in physical activity can decrease the frequency of sleep disturbances, such as insomnia or

interrupted sleep, which can exacerbate pain and fatigue.

Increased Energy Levels:

Regular exercise helps in boosting energy levels and reducing feelings of fatigue. Benefits include:

- Enhanced Stamina: Physical activity increases overall stamina and energy levels, allowing individuals to perform daily tasks with greater ease and less exhaustion.
- Reduced Fatigue: Exercise improves circulation and oxygen delivery to tissues, reducing feelings of fatigue and promoting a sense of vitality and well-being.

Emotional and Cognitive Benefits:

Stress Reduction:

Physical activity is an effective way to manage stress and anxiety, which can impact chronic pain. Benefits include:

- Stress Relief: Exercise helps in reducing stress levels by promoting the release of neurotransmitters that regulate mood and relaxation. Lower stress levels contribute to improved pain management and overall well-being.
- Cognitive Function: Regular physical activity supports cognitive function and mental clarity, which can positively affect coping strategies and pain management approaches.

Social Interaction:

Participating in group exercise or physical therapy sessions provides opportunities for social interaction, which can enhance emotional support. Benefits include:

- Social Engagement: Engaging in group activities or classes allows individuals to connect with others, share experiences, and build a support network, contributing to emotional well-being and motivation.
- Motivation and Accountability: Social interactions in exercise settings provide motivation and accountability, encouraging individuals to adhere to their exercise routines and maintain consistent efforts.

Integrating Physical Activity into Daily Routine:

Developing an Exercise Plan:

Creating a structured exercise plan tailored to individual needs and capabilities is essential for effective pain management. Key components include:

- Goal Setting: Establishing specific, achievable goals for physical activity based on personal preferences, pain levels, and functional abilities. Goals should be realistic and focus on gradual progress.
- Variety of Activities: Incorporating a variety of exercise types, such as aerobic, strength training, and flexibility exercises, to address different

aspects of physical health and manage pain effectively.

- Scheduling: Allocating regular time for physical activity within the daily routine. Consistent scheduling helps in establishing exercise habits and ensuring adherence to the plan.

Choosing Appropriate Exercises:

Selecting exercises that are suitable for individual needs and pain conditions is crucial for maximizing benefits and minimizing discomfort. Key considerations include:

- Low-Impact Activities: Choosing low-impact exercises, such as walking, swimming, or cycling, to reduce stress on joints and minimize the risk of exacerbating pain.

- Adapted Exercises: Modifying exercises to accommodate specific pain conditions or physical limitations. Adapted exercises can help in managing pain while still providing the benefits of physical activity.

Monitoring and Adjusting:

Regular monitoring of exercise progress and adjusting the plan as needed is essential for maintaining effectiveness. Key steps include:

- Tracking Progress: Keeping a record of exercise routines, pain levels, and functional improvements. Tracking progress helps in evaluating the effectiveness of the plan and making informed adjustments.

- Adjusting Intensity: Modifying the intensity, duration, or type of exercise based on changes in pain levels or physical capabilities. Adjustments ensure that the exercise plan remains appropriate and effective.

RECOMMENDED EXERCISES FOR CHRONIC PAIN

When managing chronic pain, choosing the right exercises is crucial for improving physical function, reducing pain, and enhancing overall quality of life. Certain exercises can help in managing chronic pain by focusing on flexibility, strength, and endurance while minimizing the risk of exacerbating symptoms. This section explores various types of exercises recommended for chronic pain, outlines their benefits, and provides guidance on incorporating them into a personalized exercise plan.

1. Flexibility Exercises:
Stretching:
Stretching exercises are essential for maintaining and improving flexibility, reducing muscle tension, and alleviating stiffness. Benefits include:
- Enhanced Range of Motion: Regular stretching helps to maintain and improve the range of

motion in joints and muscles, which is crucial for preventing stiffness and enhancing mobility.

- Reduced Muscle Tightness: Stretching exercises help to relieve muscle tightness and prevent discomfort caused by shortened or tense muscles.

Examples of Stretching Exercises:

- Hamstring Stretch: Sit on the floor with one leg extended and the other bent. Reach toward the toes of the extended leg while keeping your back straight. Hold for 20-30 seconds and repeat on the other side.
- Quadriceps Stretch: Stand with one hand holding onto a wall for balance. Bend one knee and bring the heel toward the buttocks. Hold the ankle with your hand and gently press the hip forward. Hold for 20-30 seconds and switch legs.
- Shoulder Stretch: Bring one arm across the body and use the opposite arm to pull it closer to the chest. Hold for 20-30 seconds and switch arms.

2. Strength Training Exercises:

Resistance Training:

Strength training exercises are vital for building muscle strength, supporting joints, and improving overall functional capacity. Benefits include:

- Muscle Support: Strengthening the muscles around affected areas helps to support joints and reduce strain, which can alleviate pain and improve stability.

- Increased Endurance: Building muscle strength enhances endurance and reduces fatigue, making daily activities easier to perform.

Examples of Resistance Training Exercises:

- Bodyweight Squats: Stand with feet shoulder-width apart and lower your body as if sitting into a chair. Keep your knees aligned with your toes and return to standing. Perform 10-15 repetitions.
- Modified Push-Ups: Start in a plank position with knees on the ground. Lower your chest toward the floor and push back up to the starting position. Perform 8-12 repetitions.
- Seated Rows: Sit on a chair or bench with a resistance band or light weights. Pull the band or weights toward your torso, keeping elbows close to your body. Perform 10-15 repetitions.

3. Aerobic Exercises:

Low-Impact Cardio:

Aerobic exercises improve cardiovascular health, enhance endurance, and help manage pain through the release of endorphins. Benefits include:

- Improved Cardiovascular Health: Aerobic exercises support heart health and overall circulation, contributing to better physical function and energy levels.

- Pain Relief: Engaging in low-impact cardio exercises stimulates the release of endorphins, which can help alleviate pain and improve mood.

Examples of Low-Impact Cardio Exercises:

- Walking: Walking at a moderate pace is a gentle yet effective form of aerobic exercise. Aim for 20-30 minutes of walking several times a week.
- Swimming: Swimming provides a full-body workout with minimal impact on joints. It is beneficial for improving cardiovascular fitness and reducing pain.
- Cycling: Using a stationary bike or riding a bicycle provides cardiovascular benefits while being easy on the joints. Aim for 20-30 minutes of cycling several times a week.

4. Balance and Stability Exercises:

Core Strengthening:

Core strengthening exercises enhance balance, stability, and overall functional capacity. Benefits include:

- Improved Balance: Strengthening the core muscles helps to stabilize the body and improve balance, which is essential for reducing the risk of falls and injuries.
- Enhanced Posture: A strong core supports proper posture and alignment, which can reduce strain on the back and other areas affected by chronic pain.

Examples of Core Strengthening Exercises:
- Pelvic Tilts: Lie on your back with knees bent and feet flat on the floor. Tighten your abdominal muscles and tilt your pelvis upward, pressing your lower back into the floor. Hold for a few seconds and relax. Perform 10-15 repetitions.
- Bird-Dog Exercise: Start on your hands and knees. Extend one arm forward and the opposite leg backward, keeping your back straight. Hold for a few seconds and return to the starting position. Perform 8-12 repetitions on each side.
- Side Plank: Lie on your side with legs extended and feet stacked. Lift your hips off the ground, supporting your body on your forearm. Hold for 20-30 seconds and switch sides.

5. Mind-Body Exercises:

Yoga and Tai Chi:

Mind-body exercises focus on the integration of physical movement, breath control, and mental relaxation. Benefits include:
- Stress Reduction: Yoga and Tai Chi help to reduce stress and promote relaxation, which can positively impact pain perception and overall well-being.
- Improved Flexibility and Balance: These practices enhance flexibility, balance, and

coordination, which can support pain management and improve functional abilities.

Examples of Mind-Body Exercises:

- Gentle Yoga: Incorporate poses such as Child's Pose, Cat-Cow Stretch, and Legs-Up-The-Wall Pose to promote relaxation, flexibility, and pain relief.
- Tai Chi: Practice Tai Chi movements such as the Tai Chi Chuan sequence or individual forms to improve balance, coordination, and stress reduction.

Incorporating Exercises into a Routine:

Creating a Balanced Exercise Plan:

To maximize the benefits of physical activity, develop a balanced exercise plan that includes a variety of exercise types. Consider the following:

- Combination of Exercises: Integrate flexibility, strength, aerobic, and balance exercises into your routine to address different aspects of physical health and pain management.
- Gradual Progression: Start with low-intensity exercises and gradually increase the duration and intensity as tolerated. This approach helps to build endurance and prevent overexertion.
- Consistency: Aim for regular exercise sessions throughout the week. Consistent physical activity

contributes to long-term improvements in pain management and overall well-being.

Adapting Exercises:
Adapt exercises based on individual needs and pain conditions. Key considerations include:
- Modifying Intensity: Adjust the intensity and duration of exercises based on current pain levels and physical capabilities. Modify exercises to reduce strain and prevent exacerbation of symptoms.
- Incorporating Rest Periods: Allow for adequate rest and recovery between exercise sessions. Rest periods help to prevent fatigue and support the body's healing process.

Consulting with Professionals:
Seek guidance from healthcare professionals, such as physical therapists or exercise specialists, to develop and implement an exercise plan tailored to individual needs. Professional guidance ensures:
- Safe and Effective Exercises: Healthcare professionals can recommend appropriate exercises and modifications based on specific pain conditions and functional limitations.
- Monitoring Progress: Regular check-ins with professionals help in assessing progress,

addressing challenges, and making necessary adjustments to the exercise plan.

DESIGNING AN EXERCISE ROUTINE

Designing an effective exercise routine for managing chronic pain requires careful planning and consideration of individual needs, capabilities, and goals. An ideal exercise routine should be comprehensive, addressing various aspects of physical health while being adaptable to changes in pain levels and physical condition. This section provides a detailed guide on how to create a personalized exercise routine that promotes pain management and overall well-being.

1. Assessing Individual Needs and Goals:
Identifying Pain Patterns and Limitations:
Before designing an exercise routine, it is essential to assess the specific characteristics of chronic pain and any physical limitations.
Key considerations include:
- Pain Location and Severity: Documenting the location, intensity, and duration of pain helps in selecting exercises that target affected areas and avoid exacerbating symptoms.
- Functional Limitations: Identifying any limitations in mobility, strength, or endurance

assists in designing exercises that accommodate these challenges and enhance overall function.

Setting Personal Goals:
Establishing clear and achievable goals is crucial for motivation and success. Goals should be specific, measurable, attainable, relevant, and time-bound (SMART). Examples of goals include:

- Improving Flexibility: Setting a goal to increase the range of motion in specific joints or muscles by a certain percentage or within a defined timeframe.
- Building Strength: Aiming to improve muscle strength in targeted areas, such as the core or legs, to enhance overall stability and support.
- Enhancing Endurance: Setting a goal to increase the duration or intensity of aerobic exercises, such as walking or cycling, to improve cardiovascular fitness and energy levels.

2. Creating a Balanced Exercise Plan:
Incorporating Various Exercise Types:
A well-rounded exercise routine should include a mix of different exercise types to address various aspects of physical health. Key components include:

- Flexibility Exercises: Incorporate stretching routines to improve flexibility and reduce muscle tension. Aim for 2-3 sessions per week, focusing on major muscle groups and affected areas.

- Strength Training: Include resistance exercises to build muscle strength and support joints. Aim for 2-3 sessions per week, with exercises targeting different muscle groups.
- Aerobic Exercise: Integrate low-impact cardiovascular activities to improve cardiovascular health and manage pain through endorphin release. Aim for 3-5 sessions per week, with varying durations and intensities.
- Balance and Stability Exercises: Add exercises to enhance balance and stability, which is crucial for preventing falls and improving functional capacity. Include these exercises 2-3 times per week.

Designing Exercise Sessions:

Each exercise session should be structured to maximize effectiveness while minimizing the risk of injury. Key elements include:

- Warm-Up: Begin each session with a 5-10 minute warm-up to prepare the body for exercise and reduce the risk of injury. Warm-up activities can include gentle stretching, light cardio, or dynamic movements.
- Main Workout: Perform the selected exercises according to the planned routine. For strength

training, include 2-3 sets of 8-12 repetitions per exercise. For aerobic exercise, aim for 20-30 minutes of continuous activity.

- Cool-Down: Conclude each session with a 5-10 minute cool-down to help the body transition back to a resting state. Include gentle stretching and relaxation techniques to reduce muscle soreness and promote recovery.

3. Adapting the Routine:

Modifying Exercises:

Adapt exercises based on current pain levels, physical capabilities, and progress. Key strategies include:

- Adjusting Intensity: Modify the intensity of exercises by reducing the weight, duration, or speed as needed. Gradually increase intensity based on tolerance and progress.
- Changing Exercise Types: Substitute exercises that may cause discomfort with alternative activities that provide similar benefits without exacerbating pain.
- Incorporating Rest Periods: Allow for adequate rest and recovery between exercise sessions to prevent overexertion and support the body's healing process.

Monitoring Progress and Making Adjustments:
Regularly assess progress and make necessary adjustments to the exercise routine. Key steps include:

- Tracking Progress: Keep a record of exercise sessions, pain levels, and functional improvements. Use this information to evaluate the effectiveness of the routine and identify areas for adjustment.
- Seeking Feedback: Consult with healthcare professionals or exercise specialists to review progress and receive recommendations for modifications or new exercises.
- Adjusting Goals: Revisit and update personal goals based on progress and changes in pain levels or physical condition. Set new goals as needed to continue improving physical health and managing pain.

4. Integrating Exercise into Daily Life:
Establishing a Routine:
Incorporate exercise into daily life by creating a consistent routine. Key strategies include:

- Scheduling: Set specific times for exercise sessions and incorporate them into the daily or weekly schedule. Consistency helps in building habits and ensuring regular participation.
- Finding Opportunities: Look for opportunities to include physical activity in daily activities, such

as walking or biking to work, taking the stairs, or participating in recreational activities.

- Making it Enjoyable: Choose exercises and activities that are enjoyable and align with personal preferences. Enjoyable activities increase motivation and adherence to the routine.

Balancing Exercise with Rest and Recovery:
Ensure a balance between exercise and rest to support overall well-being and prevent overexertion. Key considerations include:

- Rest Days: Incorporate rest days into the weekly routine to allow the body to recover and prevent fatigue. Rest days are essential for avoiding burnout and supporting long-term success.
- Active Recovery: On rest days, consider engaging in gentle activities such as walking or stretching to promote recovery and maintain flexibility.

5. Engaging in Professional Support:
Working with a Healthcare Professional:
Collaborate with healthcare professionals, such as physical therapists or exercise specialists, to design and implement an exercise routine. Professional support provides:

- Expert Guidance: Healthcare professionals can offer personalized recommendations and modifications based on specific pain conditions and functional limitations.

- Monitoring and Feedback: Regular check-ins with professionals help in assessing progress, addressing challenges, and making informed adjustments to the exercise routine.

Joining Exercise Programs or Classes:

Participating in structured exercise programs or classes can provide additional support and motivation. Options include:

- Group Exercise Classes: Join classes focused on low-impact activities, such as water aerobics or gentle yoga, to benefit from guided instruction and social support.
- Physical Therapy Programs: Enroll in physical therapy programs designed to address specific pain conditions and improve functional abilities through targeted exercises and techniques.

WORKING WITH A PHYSICAL THERAPIST

Collaborating with a physical therapist can be a pivotal component in managing chronic pain effectively. Physical therapists are trained professionals who specialize in evaluating, diagnosing, and treating physical impairments and functional limitations through tailored exercise programs, manual therapy, and other interventions. This section delves into the role of physical therapists, the benefits of working with them, and how to make the most out of this collaboration.

1. The Role of a Physical Therapist:
Assessment and Diagnosis:
Physical therapists conduct comprehensive assessments to understand the nature and extent of chronic pain and its impact on physical function. Key components include:

- Medical History Review: Physical therapists gather information about the patient's medical history, including previous injuries, surgeries, and chronic conditions. This helps in understanding the underlying causes of pain and any contributing factors.
- Physical Examination: A detailed physical examination is performed to assess pain levels, range of motion, strength, flexibility, and functional limitations. This may include specialized tests and measurements to evaluate specific impairments.
- Functional Assessment: The therapist evaluates how chronic pain affects daily activities and overall quality of life. This assessment helps in identifying specific challenges and setting appropriate treatment goals.

Creating a Personalized Treatment Plan:

Based on the assessment findings, physical therapists develop individualized treatment plans tailored to the patient's needs and goals. Key elements include:

- Exercise Prescription: Physical therapists design customized exercise programs that address specific impairments and promote functional improvements. Exercises may focus on strength, flexibility, balance, and endurance.

- Manual Therapy Techniques: Therapists may use manual therapy techniques such as joint mobilization, soft tissue manipulation, and massage to alleviate pain, reduce muscle tension, and improve joint mobility.

- Education and Self-Management: Physical therapists provide education on pain management strategies, posture, body mechanics, and activity modification. Self-management techniques empower patients to take an active role in their care.

2. Benefits of Working with a Physical Therapist:

Targeted Pain Relief:

Working with a physical therapist offers several benefits for pain management, including:

- Customized Interventions: Physical therapists tailor interventions to address the specific causes and manifestations of chronic pain, providing targeted relief and improving functional outcomes.

- Evidence-Based Approaches: Therapists utilize evidence-based practices and clinical guidelines to ensure that treatment methods are effective and supported by current research.

Improved Function and Mobility:

Collaborating with a physical therapist can lead to significant improvements in physical function and mobility:

- Enhanced Strength and Flexibility: Targeted exercises help to build muscle strength, improve flexibility, and support joint function, contributing to better overall physical capabilities.
- Increased Range of Motion: Manual therapy techniques and stretching exercises can improve the range of motion in affected joints and muscles, enhancing mobility and reducing stiffness.

Education and Empowerment:

Physical therapists provide valuable education and resources that empower patients to manage their pain and improve their quality of life:

- Pain Management Strategies: Therapists teach patients various pain management techniques, including relaxation exercises, breathing techniques, and cognitive-behavioral strategies.

- Self-Care Techniques: Patients learn self-care techniques such as proper body mechanics, ergonomic adjustments, and activity modifications to prevent pain exacerbation and promote long-term health.

3. Making the Most of Physical Therapy:

Setting Clear Goals:

Establishing clear and achievable goals is essential for maximizing the benefits of physical therapy. Key steps include:

- Defining Objectives: Work with the physical therapist to set specific, measurable, and realistic goals related to pain relief, functional improvements, and overall well-being.
- Tracking Progress: Regularly review progress toward goals with the therapist and adjust the treatment plan as needed based on progress and changes in symptoms.

Communicating Openly:

Effective communication with the physical therapist is crucial for optimizing treatment outcomes:

- Discussing Symptoms: Share detailed information about pain levels, symptoms, and any changes in condition to ensure that the treatment plan remains relevant and effective.

- Providing Feedback: Offer feedback on the effectiveness of interventions and any difficulties encountered during exercises or activities. This information helps the therapist make necessary adjustments.

Adhering to the Treatment Plan:

Consistency and adherence to the prescribed treatment plan are key factors in achieving positive outcomes:

- Following Recommendations: Adhere to the exercise program, manual therapy sessions, and any additional recommendations provided by the therapist.
- Incorporating Home Exercises: Complete any home exercise assignments as directed by the therapist to reinforce progress and support ongoing improvements.

Integrating Therapy into Daily Life:

Incorporate the skills and techniques learned during therapy into daily life to enhance long-term success:

- Applying Education: Implement pain management strategies, ergonomic adjustments, and body mechanics into daily activities to prevent pain exacerbation and support overall health.

- Maintaining Physical Activity: Continue engaging in regular physical activity and exercise beyond the therapy sessions to sustain improvements and promote overall well-being.

4. Types of Physical Therapy Interventions:

Manual Therapy:

Manual therapy involves hands-on techniques to address pain and dysfunction. Key interventions include:

- Joint Mobilization: Gentle movements applied to joints to improve mobility and reduce pain.
- Soft Tissue Mobilization: Techniques such as massage and myofascial release to alleviate muscle tension and improve circulation.
- Trigger Point Therapy: Targeted pressure applied to specific points in muscles to relieve pain and discomfort.

Exercise Therapy:

Exercise therapy focuses on improving physical function and strength through tailored exercises. Key components include:

- Strengthening Exercises: Exercises designed to build muscle strength and support affected areas.
- Stretching Exercises: Exercises to improve flexibility and reduce muscle tension.

- Functional Exercises: Activities that mimic daily tasks to improve functional capacity and mobility.

Neuromuscular Re-education:
Neuromuscular re-education involves techniques to restore normal movement patterns and improve coordination:
- Balance Training: Exercises to enhance balance and stability, reducing the risk of falls and improving functional abilities.
- Coordination Exercises: Activities to improve coordination and motor control, supporting better movement patterns.

5. Working with Insurance and Healthcare Providers:
Navigating Insurance Coverage:
Understand insurance coverage and benefits related to physical therapy to ensure access to necessary services:
- Verification of Benefits: Check with the insurance provider to confirm coverage for physical therapy services, including any limitations or requirements.
- Preauthorization: Obtain any required preauthorization for physical therapy sessions, if applicable.

Coordinating with Healthcare Providers:
Collaborate with other healthcare providers involved in your care to ensure a comprehensive approach:

- Sharing Information: Share information from physical therapy sessions with primary care physicians or specialists to ensure coordinated care and alignment with overall treatment goals.
- Integrating Treatments: Coordinate physical therapy with other treatments, such as medications or surgeries, to optimize outcomes and address all aspects of care.

CHAPTER 4

MINDFULNESS AND STRESS MANAGEMENT

INTRODUCTION TO MINDFULNESS

Mindfulness is a practice rooted in ancient traditions and modern psychological research, emphasizing present-moment awareness and acceptance. It involves paying deliberate attention to one's thoughts, feelings, and surroundings without judgment. This section explores the fundamental concepts of mindfulness, its origins, and its relevance in managing chronic pain and stress.

1. Understanding Mindfulness:
Concept of Mindfulness:
Mindfulness is a mental practice that cultivates awareness of the present moment by focusing on thoughts, emotions, bodily sensations, and the surrounding environment. This practice encourages individuals to experience each moment fully and without

distraction, promoting a deeper connection with oneself and one's environment. Key aspects include:

- Attention and Awareness: Mindfulness involves directing attention to the present moment, which helps individuals become more aware of their internal and external experiences. This heightened awareness allows for a better understanding of how thoughts, feelings, and physical sensations interact.
- Non-Judgmental Observation: A fundamental principle of mindfulness is observing experiences without judgment. This means acknowledging and accepting thoughts and feelings as they are, without labeling them as good or bad. This non-judgmental stance helps reduce self-criticism and promotes a more balanced perspective.

Historical and Cultural Context:

Mindfulness has its roots in various cultural and spiritual traditions, with notable influences from Buddhism, Hinduism, and Taoism. Each tradition offers its interpretation and practice of mindfulness:

- Buddhist Traditions: In Buddhism, mindfulness (known as "sati" in Pali) is an essential aspect of the Eightfold Path, aimed at achieving enlightenment and liberation from suffering. Buddhist mindfulness practices include meditation, ethical conduct, and mental discipline.

- Hindu Practices: In Hinduism, mindfulness is intertwined with practices such as meditation (dhyana) and yoga. These practices emphasize self-awareness and the connection between the mind and body.
- Western Adaptations: In contemporary Western contexts, mindfulness has been integrated into various therapeutic approaches, including Mindfulness-Based Stress Reduction (MBSR) and Mindfulness-Based Cognitive Therapy (MBCT). These adaptations focus on using mindfulness techniques to manage stress, anxiety, and chronic pain.

Scientific Research and Evidence:

Recent scientific research has demonstrated the effectiveness of mindfulness practices in improving mental and physical health. Key findings include:

- Reduction in Stress: Studies have shown that mindfulness can help reduce stress by promoting relaxation and reducing the body's stress response. Mindfulness practices help regulate the stress hormone cortisol and enhance the body's ability to cope with stressors.
- Improvement in Pain Management: Mindfulness-based interventions have been found

to be effective in managing chronic pain. By increasing awareness and acceptance of pain, individuals can reduce the emotional and psychological impact of pain and improve overall well-being.

- Enhanced Emotional Regulation: Mindfulness practices improve emotional regulation by increasing awareness of emotions and reducing reactivity. This helps individuals respond to challenging situations with greater calm and composure.

2. Benefits of Mindfulness:

Enhanced Self-Awareness:

Mindfulness promotes greater self-awareness by encouraging individuals to pay attention to their internal experiences. This increased self-awareness can lead to several benefits:

- Identification of Triggers: By becoming more aware of thoughts, emotions, and physical sensations, individuals can identify patterns and triggers that contribute to pain and stress. This awareness enables more effective management of these factors.

- Improved Emotional Insight: Mindfulness fosters a deeper understanding of one's emotional responses and their impact on well-being. This insight can help individuals develop healthier coping strategies and improve emotional resilience.

Stress Reduction:

One of the primary benefits of mindfulness is its ability to reduce stress. Key mechanisms include:

- Relaxation Response: Mindfulness practices, such as meditation and deep breathing, activate the body's relaxation response, counteracting the physiological effects of stress. This promotes a state of calm and reduces symptoms of stress.
- Reduced Rumination: Mindfulness helps individuals break free from cycles of rumination and worry by focusing on the present moment. This shift in focus can alleviate feelings of anxiety and stress.

Improved Pain Management:

Mindfulness can be a valuable tool in managing chronic pain by altering the perception and response to pain:

- Pain Perception: Mindfulness practices help individuals observe pain sensations without becoming overwhelmed by them. This shift in perception can reduce the intensity and impact of pain.
- Emotional Impact: By fostering acceptance and reducing emotional reactivity to pain, mindfulness can improve overall quality of life and enhance coping abilities.

3. Incorporating Mindfulness into Daily Life:

Mindfulness Meditation Practices:

Mindfulness meditation is a core practice for cultivating mindfulness. Key techniques include:

- Breath Awareness: Focusing on the breath is a fundamental mindfulness meditation practice. By paying attention to the inhale and exhale, individuals can anchor their awareness in the present moment and calm the mind.
- Body Scan: The body scan technique involves systematically focusing on different areas of the body, observing sensations without judgment. This practice helps increase body awareness and relaxation.
- Mindful Observation: Mindful observation involves paying attention to sensory experiences, such as sights, sounds, and smells. This practice encourages full engagement with the present moment and enhances sensory awareness.

Integrating Mindfulness into Daily Activities:

Mindfulness can be incorporated into various daily activities to enhance overall well-being:

- Mindful Eating: Practicing mindful eating involves paying attention to the sensory experience of eating, such as taste, texture, and aroma. This practice promotes healthier eating habits and improves digestion.

- Mindful Walking: Mindful walking involves focusing on the physical sensations of walking, such as the movement of the legs and the feeling of the ground beneath the feet. This practice can be a calming and grounding experience.
- Mindful Communication: Practicing mindful communication involves being fully present during conversations, listening attentively, and responding thoughtfully. This practice can improve relationships and reduce interpersonal stress.

4. Overcoming Challenges in Mindfulness Practice:
Dealing with Distractions:
Distractions are a common challenge in mindfulness practice. Strategies for managing distractions include:

- Acknowledging and Letting Go: When distractions arise, acknowledge them without judgment and gently bring your focus back to the present moment. This practice helps reduce frustration and maintain mindfulness.
- Setting a Routine: Establishing a regular mindfulness practice routine can help reduce distractions and increase the likelihood of maintaining focus. Consistent practice builds familiarity and reinforces mindfulness skills.

Managing Expectations:

It is important to approach mindfulness with realistic expectations and a patient mindset:

- Acceptance of Imperfection: Mindfulness practice is not about achieving perfection but about cultivating awareness and acceptance. Embrace the process and recognize that progress may come gradually.
- Patience and Persistence: Developing mindfulness skills takes time and practice. Be patient with yourself and persist in your efforts, even if progress feels slow.

5. Seeking Support and Resources:

Mindfulness Programs and Classes:

Participating in mindfulness programs or classes can provide additional support and guidance:

- Mindfulness-Based Stress Reduction (MBSR): MBSR is a structured program that combines mindfulness meditation with yoga and stress management techniques. It is designed to help individuals manage stress and improve overall well-being.
- Mindfulness-Based Cognitive Therapy (MBCT): MBCT integrates mindfulness practices with cognitive therapy techniques to address negative thought patterns and improve emotional regulation.

Online Resources and Apps:

Numerous online resources and mobile apps offer guided mindfulness practices and support:

- Guided Meditations: Explore guided meditation apps or websites that provide audio or video instructions for various mindfulness practices, such as breath awareness or body scans.
- Mindfulness Journals: Use mindfulness journals to track your practice, reflect on experiences, and set goals. Journals can provide valuable insights and reinforce mindfulness skills.

Professional Guidance:

Consider seeking guidance from mindfulness practitioners or therapists for personalized support:

- Mindfulness Coaches: Mindfulness coaches offer individual or group sessions to teach and support mindfulness practices. They can provide tailored guidance and address specific challenges.
- Therapists with Mindfulness Training: Therapists with mindfulness training can incorporate mindfulness techniques into therapeutic sessions to address chronic pain, stress, and other concerns.

TECHNIQUES FOR STRESS REDUCTION

Stress reduction techniques are essential tools for managing both acute and chronic stress, contributing to improved mental and physical health. This section explores a variety of effective techniques for reducing stress, including their mechanisms, benefits, and practical applications.

1. Deep Breathing Exercises:

Mechanism and Benefits:

Deep breathing exercises focus on controlling the breath to activate the body's relaxation response. The process involves taking slow, deep breaths to lower heart rate and reduce stress hormones, such as cortisol.

- Diaphragmatic Breathing: This technique involves breathing deeply into the diaphragm rather than shallowly into the chest. It promotes better oxygenation, activates the parasympathetic nervous system, and induces a calming effect. Diaphragmatic breathing helps reduce anxiety and improve overall relaxation.
- 4-7-8 Breathing: The 4-7-8 breathing technique involves inhaling for 4 seconds, holding the breath for 7 seconds, and exhaling slowly for 8 seconds. This method promotes relaxation by slowing down the breath and focusing attention, which can help manage stress and improve sleep.
- Box Breathing: Box breathing consists of inhaling for 4 seconds, holding the breath for 4 seconds, exhaling for 4 seconds, and holding the breath again for 4 seconds. This technique helps

regulate the breath and calm the mind, making it useful for reducing stress and enhancing focus.

Practical Applications:

- Daily Practice: Integrate deep breathing exercises into daily routines, such as during work breaks or before bedtime. Short, frequent sessions can enhance overall stress management.
- Stressful Situations: Use deep breathing techniques during high-stress situations, such as presentations or conflicts, to maintain composure and reduce immediate stress.

2. Progressive Muscle Relaxation (PMR):

Mechanism and Benefits:

Progressive Muscle Relaxation (PMR) involves tensing and then relaxing different muscle groups to reduce physical tension and stress. By becoming aware of muscle tension and consciously relaxing it, individuals can alleviate stress-related symptoms.

- Muscle Tension Awareness: PMR helps individuals identify areas of muscle tension and understand how stress affects the body. By focusing on relaxation, individuals can release accumulated tension and promote physical relaxation.
- Stress Relief: Regular PMR practice can reduce overall stress levels, lower blood pressure, and improve sleep quality. It is particularly effective

for managing physical symptoms of stress, such as muscle pain and headaches.

Practical Applications:

- Guided Sessions: Start with guided PMR sessions, available through apps or online resources, to learn the technique and ensure proper execution. Over time, practice PMR independently to enhance relaxation skills.
- Pre-Sleep Routine: Incorporate PMR into a pre-sleep routine to promote relaxation and improve sleep quality. Practicing PMR before bedtime can help reduce insomnia and enhance overall restfulness.

3. Mindfulness Meditation:

Mechanism and Benefits:

Mindfulness meditation involves focusing on the present moment and cultivating awareness without judgment. This practice helps manage stress by promoting relaxation, increasing self-awareness, and reducing emotional reactivity.

- Present-Moment Awareness: Mindfulness meditation encourages individuals to observe their thoughts, emotions, and sensations without becoming overwhelmed by them. This practice fosters a sense of calm and detachment from stressors.
- Reduction of Stress Responses: Regular mindfulness meditation can reduce the body's

stress response, lower cortisol levels, and improve overall emotional regulation. It helps individuals develop a more balanced perspective on stressors.

Practical Applications:

- Daily Practice: Set aside time each day for mindfulness meditation, starting with short sessions and gradually increasing duration. Consistent practice can enhance stress management and overall well-being.
- Mindfulness Integration: Integrate mindfulness techniques into daily activities, such as eating or walking, to cultivate a mindful approach to life and manage stress in real-time.

4. Visualization Techniques:

Mechanism and Benefits:

Visualization techniques involve imagining peaceful or positive scenarios to reduce stress and promote relaxation. By engaging the mind in calming imagery, individuals can experience reduced stress and improved emotional well-being.

- Guided Imagery: Guided imagery involves listening to verbal instructions that lead individuals through calming visualizations, such as imagining a serene beach or a peaceful forest. This practice helps create a mental escape from stress and promotes relaxation.

- Self-Guided Visualization: Self-guided visualization allows individuals to create their own calming mental images and scenarios. This technique can be tailored to personal preferences and needs, enhancing its effectiveness.

Practical Applications:

- Stressful Situations: Use visualization techniques during stressful moments, such as before a challenging meeting or exam, to create a sense of calm and boost confidence.
- Daily Practice: Incorporate visualization exercises into a daily relaxation routine, such as before bedtime or during breaks, to maintain a sense of calm and reduce overall stress.

5. Yoga and Stretching:

Mechanism and Benefits:

Yoga and stretching combine physical movement with breath control and mindfulness to reduce stress and promote relaxation. These practices help improve flexibility, balance, and overall physical and mental well-being.

- Yoga Practice: Yoga involves a series of postures and breathing exercises that promote relaxation, improve flexibility, and reduce physical tension. It enhances the mind-body connection and supports stress management through mindful movement and deep breathing.

- Stretching: Stretching exercises target specific muscle groups to alleviate physical tension and improve circulation. Regular stretching helps release muscle tightness and contributes to overall relaxation.

Practical Applications:

- Yoga Classes: Join yoga classes or follow online tutorials to learn and practice various yoga poses and techniques. Choose classes that focus on relaxation and stress reduction for optimal benefits.

- Home Practice: Incorporate yoga and stretching into a home exercise routine, using online resources or instructional videos. Regular practice can enhance stress management and promote physical well-being.

6. Cognitive-Behavioral Techniques:

Mechanism and Benefits:

Cognitive-behavioral techniques focus on changing negative thought patterns and behaviors that contribute to stress. By addressing cognitive distortions and promoting positive thinking, individuals can manage stress more effectively.

- Cognitive Restructuring: Cognitive restructuring involves identifying and challenging negative or irrational thoughts and replacing them with more balanced and positive thoughts. This technique helps reduce stress and improve emotional well-being.

- Behavioral Activation: Behavioral activation involves engaging in activities that bring pleasure and satisfaction to counteract feelings of stress and depression. By focusing on enjoyable activities, individuals can improve mood and reduce stress.

Practical Applications:

- Therapeutic Sessions: Work with a cognitive-behavioral therapist to learn and apply cognitive-behavioral techniques for stress management. Therapy can provide personalized strategies and support for addressing specific stressors.
- Self-Help Resources: Utilize self-help books or online resources that focus on cognitive-behavioral techniques for stress reduction. These resources can provide valuable insights and practical exercises for managing stress.

7. Social Support and Connection:

Mechanism and Benefits:

Social support and connection involve seeking and maintaining relationships with family, friends, and support networks to manage stress and enhance well-being. Social interactions provide emotional support, practical assistance, and a sense of belonging.

- Emotional Support: Engaging with supportive individuals can provide emotional relief and reduce feelings of isolation. Sharing concerns and receiving empathy from others helps alleviate stress and enhances emotional resilience.
- Practical Assistance: Social support can offer practical help in managing stress, such as assistance with daily tasks or problem-solving. Supportive networks contribute to overall stress management and well-being.

Practical Applications:

- Building Relationships: Cultivate and maintain meaningful relationships with family, friends, and community members. Engage in regular social activities and seek support when needed.
- Support Groups: Participate in support groups or online communities that focus on specific stressors or challenges. These groups provide opportunities for sharing experiences, gaining insights, and receiving support from others.

INCORPORATING MINDFULNESS INTO DAILY LIFE

Incorporating mindfulness into daily life involves integrating mindful practices into routine activities to enhance overall well-being and manage stress. Mindfulness is the practice of paying full attention to the present moment without judgment, and it can be applied to various aspects of daily living to improve mental and emotional health. This section explores practical strategies for embedding mindfulness into everyday activities, including the benefits and techniques for doing so effectively.

1. Mindful Eating:
Concept and Benefits:
Mindful eating involves paying close attention to the experience of eating, including the taste, texture, and aroma of food, as well as recognizing hunger and satiety cues. This practice encourages a more intentional and aware approach to eating, promoting healthier relationships with food and better digestion.

- Awareness of Sensations: By focusing on the sensory experience of eating, individuals can develop a deeper appreciation for their meals and make more conscious choices about portion sizes and food quality. This practice helps prevent overeating and promotes healthier eating habits.

- Emotional Connection: Mindful eating helps individuals recognize emotional triggers for eating and address emotional eating patterns. By being present with food, individuals can better understand their motivations and improve their overall relationship with eating.

Practical Applications:

- Slow Down: Take time to savor each bite, chew slowly, and appreciate the flavors and textures of the food. Avoid distractions such as television or smartphones during meals to enhance focus on the eating experience.
- Check-In with Hunger: Before eating, assess your level of hunger and eat only until you feel satisfied. Practice mindful eating by paying attention to how your body feels before, during, and after meals.

2. Mindful Commuting:

Concept and Benefits:

Mindful commuting involves practicing mindfulness during travel to reduce stress and enhance the commuting experience. This approach encourages a calm and present mindset while navigating daily transportation routines, whether by car, public transit, or walking.

- Stress Reduction: Mindful commuting helps manage the stress often associated with traffic, delays, or crowded public transportation. By staying present and focused, individuals can reduce anxiety and enhance their overall sense of calm.

- Enhanced Enjoyment: Practicing mindfulness during commuting allows individuals to appreciate the journey and find moments of relaxation or inspiration. This approach can transform commuting from a stressful chore into a more enjoyable and peaceful experience.

Practical Applications:

- Focused Breathing: Use commute time to practice deep breathing or mindfulness exercises. For example, focus on your breath while driving or listen to guided mindfulness meditations during public transit.
- Present-Moment Awareness: Pay attention to the sights, sounds, and sensations of your commute. Observe the environment with curiosity and engage in mindful listening or observation to stay grounded in the present moment.

3. Mindful Work Habits:

Concept and Benefits:

Incorporating mindfulness into work habits can enhance productivity, reduce stress, and improve overall job satisfaction. Mindful work practices involve being fully present and engaged in work tasks, fostering a more focused and less reactive approach to challenges.

- Improved Concentration: Mindfulness helps individuals stay focused on the task at hand, reducing distractions and enhancing concentration. This leads to more efficient work and higher-quality outcomes.
- Stress Management: By practicing mindfulness, individuals can manage work-related stress more effectively, respond calmly to challenges, and maintain a balanced perspective on job demands.

Practical Applications:

- Mindful Breaks: Take short, mindful breaks throughout the workday to reset and recharge. Use these breaks to engage in mindful breathing, stretching, or brief meditation to alleviate stress and enhance focus.
- Intentional Task Management: Approach work tasks with mindfulness by setting clear intentions, prioritizing tasks, and focusing fully on one task at a time. Avoid multitasking and manage distractions to improve work efficiency and satisfaction.

4. Mindful Communication:

Concept and Benefits:

Mindful communication involves being fully present and attentive during interactions with others. This practice enhances the quality of communication, fosters better relationships, and reduces misunderstandings and conflicts.

- Active Listening: Mindful communication emphasizes active listening, where individuals fully concentrate on what the other person is saying without interrupting or planning their response. This approach promotes deeper understanding and empathy in conversations.
- Thoughtful Responses: Practicing mindfulness in communication helps individuals respond thoughtfully rather than reacting impulsively. This leads to more effective and respectful interactions and reduces the likelihood of conflicts.

Practical Applications:

- Mindful Presence: During conversations, give your full attention to the speaker, maintain eye contact, and avoid distractions such as checking your phone or thinking about your response.
- Pause Before Responding: Take a moment to pause and reflect before responding to ensure your reply is considered and relevant. This practice promotes more meaningful and respectful communication.

5. Mindful Relaxation:

Concept and Benefits:

Mindful relaxation involves integrating mindfulness into relaxation practices to enhance their effectiveness. This approach combines mindfulness with activities such as reading, taking a bath, or listening to music to promote relaxation and stress relief.

- Enhanced Relaxation: By practicing mindfulness during relaxation activities, individuals can deepen their sense of relaxation and enjoyment. This practice helps to fully engage in the activity and release stress more effectively.
- Stress Relief: Mindful relaxation techniques contribute to overall stress management by promoting a sense of calm and reducing the impact of stressors on daily life.

Practical Applications:

- Mindful Leisure: Engage in leisure activities with full attention and presence. Whether reading a book, enjoying a bath, or listening to music, focus on the sensory experience and allow yourself to fully relax.
- Relaxation Routine: Incorporate mindful relaxation into a regular routine, such as before bedtime or during breaks, to maintain a sense of calm and enhance overall well-being.

6. Mindful Technology Use:

Concept and Benefits:

Mindful technology use involves applying mindfulness principles to the use of digital devices and online interactions. This practice helps manage technology-related stress, improve digital well-being, and enhance overall mindfulness.

- Reduced Digital Stress: By practicing mindfulness with technology, individuals can manage digital distractions, avoid information overload, and maintain a healthier relationship with digital devices.
- Enhanced Focus: Mindful technology use promotes intentional and focused interactions with digital content, reducing multitasking and improving overall productivity and satisfaction.

Practical Applications:

- Digital Detox: Set boundaries for technology use, such as designated times for checking emails or social media. Practice mindful use by focusing on one task or interaction at a time.
- Mindful Scrolling: Pay attention to your digital interactions, such as social media scrolling or email reading. Notice how these activities impact your mood and well-being, and adjust your habits accordingly.

THE ROLE OF MEDITATION AND BREATHING EXERCISES

Meditation and breathing exercises are fundamental components of mindfulness practices that play a crucial role in managing stress and enhancing overall well-being. Both techniques offer unique benefits and can be integrated into daily routines to support mental, emotional, and physical health. This section delves into the principles, techniques, and benefits of meditation and breathing exercises, providing a comprehensive understanding of how these practices can be effectively used to improve quality of life.

Meditation

Concept and Benefits:

Meditation is a practice that involves focusing the mind and calming the body to achieve a state of mental clarity and relaxation. It encompasses various techniques that aim to enhance awareness, reduce stress, and promote overall well-being.

- Enhanced Focus and Clarity: Regular meditation practice helps sharpen concentration and mental clarity. By training the mind to focus on a single point of attention, such as the breath or a mantra, individuals can improve their ability to concentrate and reduce mental clutter.
- Stress Reduction: Meditation has been shown to lower levels of stress hormones, such as cortisol. By promoting relaxation and fostering a sense of calm, meditation helps manage stress and anxiety, contributing to overall emotional stability.
- Emotional Regulation: Meditation encourages the development of emotional resilience and balance.

It helps individuals observe their thoughts and emotions without judgment, leading to greater self-awareness and improved emotional regulation.

Techniques:

1. Mindfulness Meditation:

   - Practice: In mindfulness meditation, individuals focus on the present moment by paying attention to their breath, bodily sensations, or surrounding environment. The goal is to observe thoughts and feelings without attachment or judgment.

   - Application: This technique can be practiced in various settings, such as sitting quietly or engaging in mindful activities like walking or eating.

2. Loving-Kindness Meditation (Metta):

   - Practice: Loving-kindness meditation involves silently repeating phrases of goodwill and compassion towards oneself and others. It aims to cultivate feelings of love, kindness, and empathy.

   - Application: This practice helps foster positive emotions and improve relationships by promoting a compassionate mindset.

3. Body Scan Meditation:

   - Practice: In body scan meditation, individuals systematically focus on different parts of the body, noticing sensations and releasing tension.

This technique enhances body awareness and relaxation.

- Application: Body scan meditation is often used to address physical discomfort or stress, promoting a deeper connection between mind and body.

4. Guided Meditation:

- Practice: Guided meditation involves listening to a narrator or recording that provides instructions and imagery to guide the meditation experience. It helps individuals relax and focus by following verbal cues.

- Application: Guided meditation is beneficial for beginners or those seeking specific themes, such as relaxation, stress relief, or sleep.

Breathing Exercises

Concept and Benefits:

Breathing exercises involve conscious control of the breath to achieve relaxation and mental clarity. These exercises can regulate physiological responses and influence emotional states, offering numerous health benefits.

- Improved Oxygenation: Deep and controlled breathing enhances oxygen delivery to the body's cells, improving overall energy levels and supporting physical health.

- Stress Reduction: Breathing exercises help activate the parasympathetic nervous system, which counteracts the stress response and promotes relaxation. This leads to a reduction in anxiety and a sense of calm.

- Enhanced Focus and Mental Clarity: Controlled breathing techniques can improve concentration and mental clarity by calming the mind and reducing distractions.

Techniques:

1. Diaphragmatic Breathing:
   - Practice: Diaphragmatic breathing involves engaging the diaphragm to take deep breaths. Individuals breathe deeply through the nose, allowing the abdomen to rise, and exhale slowly through the mouth.
   - Application: This technique helps promote relaxation and can be practiced in various situations, such as during stress or before sleep.

2. Box Breathing:
   - Practice: Box breathing involves inhaling, holding, exhaling, and pausing for equal counts, typically four seconds each. This structured breathing pattern helps regulate the breath and calm the nervous system.
   - Application: Box breathing is effective for managing acute stress or anxiety and

can be used during moments of high tension or in daily practice.

3. 4-7-8 Breathing:
   - o Practice: In 4-7-8 breathing, individuals inhale through the nose for four seconds, hold the breath for seven seconds, and exhale through the mouth for eight seconds. This technique promotes relaxation and improves sleep quality.
   - o Application: 4-7-8 breathing is beneficial for managing stress, improving sleep, and calming the mind before bedtime.
4. Alternate Nostril Breathing:
   - o Practice: Alternate nostril breathing involves closing one nostril while inhaling through the other, then switching nostrils and exhaling. This technique balances the nervous system and enhances mental clarity.
   - o Application: Alternate nostril breathing can be practiced to reduce stress and promote a sense of balance and calm.

Integrating Meditation and Breathing Exercises into Daily Life

Incorporating meditation and breathing exercises into daily routines enhances overall well-being and supports effective stress management. Practical strategies for integrating these practices include:

- Designate Time: Set aside specific times for meditation and breathing exercises, such as in the morning or before bedtime. Consistent practice helps establish a routine and reinforces the benefits.
- Create a Space: Designate a quiet and comfortable space for meditation and breathing exercises. A dedicated space enhances focus and encourages regular practice.
- Use Technology: Utilize meditation apps or online resources to access guided meditations and breathing exercises. These tools provide structure and support for developing a regular practice.
- Combine with Other Practices: Integrate meditation and breathing exercises with other mindfulness practices, such as mindful eating or mindful walking, to enhance overall mindfulness and well-being.

CHAPTER 5

NUTRITION AND DIET ADJUSTMENTS

IMPACT OF DIET ON CHRONIC PAIN

The relationship between diet and chronic pain is complex and multifaceted, involving a range of physiological, biochemical, and inflammatory processes. Understanding how dietary choices influence chronic pain can empower individuals to make informed nutritional adjustments that may alleviate symptoms and improve overall well-being. This section explores the various ways in which diet affects chronic pain, including the role of inflammation, nutrient deficiencies, and the impact of specific dietary components.

1. Inflammation and Chronic Pain:
Concept and Mechanisms:
Inflammation is a key factor in many chronic pain conditions, such as arthritis, fibromyalgia, and chronic back pain. Certain foods can either exacerbate or alleviate inflammation, influencing pain levels and overall health.

- Pro-inflammatory Foods: Diets high in refined sugars, saturated fats, and processed foods can contribute to chronic inflammation. These foods can increase the production of pro-inflammatory cytokines and oxidative stress, which can aggravate pain conditions.

- Anti-inflammatory Foods: Conversely, diets rich in anti-inflammatory foods can help reduce inflammation and alleviate pain. Foods high in omega-3 fatty acids, antioxidants, and fiber have been shown to have anti-inflammatory effects and support overall health.

Practical Dietary Adjustments:

- Incorporate Omega-3 Fatty Acids: Omega-3 fatty acids, found in fatty fish (e.g., salmon, mackerel), flaxseeds, and walnuts, have been shown to reduce inflammation and may help alleviate chronic pain.
- Increase Antioxidant-Rich Foods: Foods rich in antioxidants, such as fruits (e.g., berries, cherries) and vegetables (e.g., spinach, kale), can combat oxidative stress and inflammation. Incorporating these foods into the diet may support pain management.
- Limit Processed and Sugary Foods: Reducing the intake of processed foods, sugary snacks, and high-fat foods can help decrease inflammation and improve pain symptoms. Focus on whole, unprocessed foods for better health outcomes.

2. Nutrient Deficiencies and Pain Management:

Concept and Impact:

Nutrient deficiencies can exacerbate chronic pain by impairing various bodily functions, including immune response, tissue repair, and pain modulation. Ensuring adequate intake of essential nutrients can support pain management and overall health.

- Vitamin D: Vitamin D deficiency is associated with increased pain sensitivity and may contribute to conditions such as fibromyalgia. Ensuring adequate vitamin D levels through sunlight exposure, dietary sources, or supplements can help manage pain.
- Magnesium: Magnesium plays a role in muscle function and nerve transmission. Deficiency in magnesium may lead to muscle cramps and increased pain sensitivity. Foods rich in magnesium, such as leafy greens, nuts, and seeds, can support pain management.
- B Vitamins: B vitamins, particularly B12 and B6, are important for nerve health and pain perception. Deficiencies in these vitamins can lead to neuropathic pain. Including foods rich in B vitamins, such as eggs, dairy products, and fortified cereals, can be beneficial.

Practical Dietary Adjustments:

- Ensure Adequate Vitamin D Intake: Incorporate vitamin D-rich foods like fatty fish, fortified dairy products, and egg yolks. Consider vitamin

D supplementation if levels are low, as advised by a healthcare provider.

- Boost Magnesium Intake: Increase dietary magnesium by consuming foods such as almonds, pumpkin seeds, and spinach. Magnesium supplements may be considered under the guidance of a healthcare professional.
- Maintain B Vitamin Levels: Consume a varied diet that includes sources of B vitamins, such as lean meats, whole grains, and legumes. Consider a B-complex supplement if deficiencies are identified.

3. Special Diets and Chronic Pain:

Concept and Benefits:

Certain dietary patterns and special diets have been investigated for their potential to manage chronic pain. These diets focus on specific food groups or elimination strategies to address pain and inflammation.

- Mediterranean Diet: The Mediterranean diet, rich in fruits, vegetables, whole grains, and healthy fats (e.g., olive oil), has been associated with reduced inflammation and improved pain outcomes. Its emphasis on nutrient-dense foods and healthy fats supports overall health.
- Anti-inflammatory Diet: An anti-inflammatory diet focuses on foods that reduce inflammation, such as fatty fish, nuts, and whole grains, while avoiding pro-inflammatory foods like processed

meats and sugary beverages. This diet aims to alleviate pain and improve quality of life.

- Elimination Diets: Elimination diets involve removing specific food groups (e.g., gluten, dairy) to identify potential triggers for pain and inflammation. These diets can help individuals pinpoint foods that may contribute to their symptoms and make necessary adjustments.

Practical Dietary Adjustments:

- Adopt a Mediterranean Diet: Incorporate more fruits, vegetables, whole grains, and healthy fats into daily meals. Emphasize plant-based foods and limit red meat and processed foods.

- Follow an Anti-inflammatory Diet: Focus on anti-inflammatory foods, such as fatty fish, nuts, and leafy greens, while avoiding processed and high-sugar foods. Tailor the diet to individual preferences and needs.

- Implement Elimination Diets Carefully: If considering an elimination diet, do so under the guidance of a healthcare provider or nutritionist. Monitor symptoms and make gradual adjustments to identify potential food triggers.

4. Hydration and Pain Management:

Concept and Importance:

Adequate hydration is essential for overall health and can influence chronic pain. Dehydration can exacerbate pain and discomfort by affecting bodily functions and increasing muscle tension.

- Hydration and Muscle Function: Proper hydration supports muscle function and reduces the risk of cramps and stiffness. Dehydration can lead to increased muscle pain and reduced flexibility.
- Joint Health: Staying hydrated helps maintain joint lubrication and cartilage health. Dehydration can contribute to joint stiffness and discomfort, potentially exacerbating pain conditions.

Practical Dietary Adjustments:

- Maintain Hydration: Aim to drink sufficient water throughout the day, based on individual needs and activity levels. Consider increasing fluid intake if engaging in physical activity or experiencing hot weather.
- Incorporate Hydrating Foods: Include water-rich foods, such as fruits (e.g., watermelon, oranges) and vegetables (e.g., cucumber, celery), to support hydration and overall health.

ANTI-INFLAMMATORY FOODS

Anti-inflammatory foods are key to managing chronic pain and promoting overall health. They help reduce inflammation, which is often a major contributor to chronic pain conditions such as arthritis, fibromyalgia, and back pain. This section explores various anti-inflammatory foods, their mechanisms of action, and practical ways to incorporate them into your diet for optimal benefits.

1. Fruits and Vegetables

Concept and Benefits:

Fruits and vegetables are rich in vitamins, minerals, and antioxidants that combat inflammation. Their high content of phytonutrients, fiber, and essential vitamins helps reduce oxidative stress and support the body's anti-inflammatory processes.

- Berries: Berries such as blueberries, strawberries, and raspberries are packed with antioxidants like anthocyanins and flavonoids, which help neutralize free radicals and reduce inflammation. Studies suggest that consuming berries regularly can lower markers of inflammation and improve overall health.

- Leafy Greens: Vegetables like spinach, kale, and Swiss chard are high in vitamins A, C, and K, as well as antioxidants such as lutein and zeaxanthin. These nutrients play a role in reducing inflammation and supporting immune function.

- Cruciferous Vegetables: Vegetables such as broccoli, Brussels sprouts, and cauliflower contain sulforaphane, a compound with potent anti-inflammatory properties. They also provide essential nutrients like vitamin C and fiber.

Practical Dietary Adjustments:

- Include a Variety of Fruits and Vegetables: Aim to incorporate a range of colorful fruits and vegetables into your meals. Fresh or frozen berries can be added to smoothies, yogurt, or cereals, while leafy greens and cruciferous vegetables can be included in salads, stir-fries, and soups.

- Experiment with Different Preparations: Enjoy fruits and vegetables in various forms, such as raw, steamed, roasted, or blended, to keep your diet interesting and maximize nutrient intake.

2. Fatty Fish

Concept and Benefits:

Fatty fish are an excellent source of omega-3 fatty acids, which are known for their anti-inflammatory effects. Omega-3s help reduce the production of inflammatory cytokines and prostaglandins, contributing to decreased pain and improved joint health.

- Salmon: Rich in EPA and DHA, two types of omega-3 fatty acids, salmon is known for its powerful anti-inflammatory properties. Consuming salmon regularly can help lower inflammation and support cardiovascular health.

- Mackerel: Another fatty fish high in omega-3s, mackerel is also a good source of vitamin D.

Regular consumption of mackerel can contribute to reduced inflammation and improved bone health.

- Sardines: Sardines are not only rich in omega-3s but also provide calcium and vitamin D. They are a convenient and affordable option for reducing inflammation and supporting overall health.

Practical Dietary Adjustments:

- Incorporate Fatty Fish into Meals: Aim to include fatty fish in your diet at least two to three times a week. Enjoy grilled, baked, or broiled fish, and consider using fish oil supplements if fresh fish is not available.
- Explore Various Recipes: Experiment with different recipes to include fatty fish in your diet, such as fish tacos, salmon patties, or mackerel salads.

3. Nuts and Seeds

Concept and Benefits:

Nuts and seeds are rich in healthy fats, fiber, and antioxidants, all of which contribute to their anti-inflammatory effects. They provide essential nutrients that support overall health and help manage chronic pain.

- Almonds: Almonds are high in monounsaturated fats and vitamin E, both of which have anti-inflammatory properties. Regular consumption of almonds can help reduce oxidative stress and support heart health.

- Chia Seeds: Chia seeds are an excellent source of omega-3 fatty acids, fiber, and antioxidants. They help reduce inflammation and improve digestive health.
- Flaxseeds: Flaxseeds contain alpha-linolenic acid (ALA), a type of omega-3 fatty acid, as well as lignans and fiber. These components contribute to reduced inflammation and improved overall health.

Practical Dietary Adjustments:

- Add Nuts and Seeds to Meals: Incorporate a variety of nuts and seeds into your diet by adding them to salads, yogurt, smoothies, or oatmeal. Almonds can be enjoyed as a snack, while chia and flaxseeds can be added to smoothies or used as egg substitutes in baking.
- Choose Unsalted and Raw Options: Opt for unsalted and raw or lightly roasted nuts and seeds to avoid added sodium and preservatives.

4. Whole Grains

Concept and Benefits:

Whole grains provide essential nutrients, including fiber, vitamins, and minerals, that contribute to their anti-inflammatory effects. Unlike refined grains, whole grains are less likely to spike blood sugar levels and contribute to inflammation.

- Quinoa: Quinoa is a complete protein and a good source of fiber, magnesium, and antioxidants. It helps regulate blood sugar levels and supports digestive health.
- Oats: Oats are high in soluble fiber, particularly beta-glucan, which helps reduce inflammation and improve cholesterol levels. They also provide essential vitamins and minerals.
- Brown Rice: Brown rice is a whole grain that provides fiber, B vitamins, and minerals. It supports digestive health and helps maintain stable blood sugar levels.

Practical Dietary Adjustments:

- Replace Refined Grains with Whole Grains: Choose whole grains such as quinoa, oats, and brown rice instead of refined grains. Use whole grain options in place of white rice, white bread, and regular pasta.
- Experiment with Whole Grain Recipes: Incorporate whole grains into a variety of dishes, such as salads, soups, and stir-fries.

5. Herbs and Spices

Concept and Benefits:

Herbs and spices are not only used for flavoring but also have anti-inflammatory properties that can help manage chronic pain. They contain bioactive compounds that support immune function and reduce inflammation.

- Turmeric: Curcumin, the active compound in turmeric, has strong anti-inflammatory and antioxidant effects. It helps reduce the production of inflammatory cytokines and supports joint health.
- Ginger: Ginger contains gingerol, a compound with anti-inflammatory and antioxidant properties. It helps alleviate pain and discomfort associated with inflammation.
- Garlic: Garlic has been shown to reduce inflammation and support cardiovascular health. Its compounds, such as allicin, have anti-inflammatory effects and contribute to overall well-being.

Practical Dietary Adjustments:

- Incorporate Herbs and Spices into Meals: Use turmeric, ginger, and garlic in cooking to add flavor and reap their anti-inflammatory benefits. Add turmeric to curries, ginger to teas or stir-fries, and garlic to various dishes.
- Experiment with Spice Blends: Create spice blends that include anti-inflammatory herbs and spices to enhance the flavor and health benefits of your meals.

FOODS TO AVOID

Avoiding certain foods is crucial in managing chronic pain and reducing inflammation. While some foods exacerbate inflammation and contribute to chronic pain, others can worsen symptoms by affecting overall health. This section explores various types of foods to avoid, their impact on chronic pain, and practical strategies for making healthier dietary choices.

1. Refined Sugars and Sweetened Beverages

Concept and Impact:

Refined sugars and sweetened beverages are known to contribute to chronic inflammation and pain. High sugar intake can lead to increased production of inflammatory cytokines and exacerbate pain conditions.

- Mechanisms of Inflammation: Refined sugars, such as those found in sugary snacks, sodas, and desserts, can cause spikes in blood glucose levels. This results in increased insulin production, which can lead to systemic inflammation and oxidative stress.

- Health Implications: Excessive sugar consumption is associated with various health issues, including obesity, metabolic syndrome, and type 2 diabetes. These conditions are linked to chronic inflammation and can exacerbate pain symptoms.

Practical Dietary Adjustments:

- Limit Added Sugars: Reduce the intake of foods and beverages with high added sugar content, such as candies, cookies, cakes, and sugary drinks. Check nutrition labels for hidden sugars in processed foods.
- Choose Natural Sweeteners: Opt for natural sweeteners like stevia or monk fruit when needed, and use them in moderation. Additionally, incorporate naturally sweet foods such as fruits in place of sugary snacks.

2. Processed and Fast Foods

Concept and Impact:

Processed and fast foods are often high in unhealthy fats, salt, and artificial additives, all of which can contribute to inflammation and worsen chronic pain.

- Unhealthy Fats: Many processed and fast foods contain trans fats and saturated fats, which have been linked to increased inflammation and cardiovascular issues. These fats are often found in fried foods, baked goods, and packaged snacks.
- High Sodium Content: Excessive sodium intake from processed foods can lead to fluid retention and increased blood pressure, exacerbating pain and discomfort. High sodium levels can also contribute to systemic inflammation.

Practical Dietary Adjustments:

- Reduce Processed Food Intake: Minimize the consumption of processed and fast foods, such as chips, frozen meals, and fast food items. Prepare meals from fresh, whole ingredients to better control the nutritional content.
- Opt for Healthier Cooking Methods: Choose cooking methods that require less oil and fat, such as baking, grilling, or steaming, instead of frying. Use herbs and spices for flavoring rather than salt.

3. Red and Processed Meats

Concept and Impact:

Red and processed meats have been linked to increased inflammation and chronic pain. These meats often contain high levels of saturated fats and compounds that can contribute to systemic inflammation.

- Saturated Fats: Red meats, such as beef and pork, are high in saturated fats, which can promote inflammation and negatively impact cardiovascular health. Processed meats, such as sausages and bacon, contain additional preservatives and additives that may exacerbate inflammation.
- Health Risks: High consumption of red and processed meats has been associated with various health problems, including heart disease, diabetes, and certain cancers. These conditions

are related to chronic inflammation and can worsen pain symptoms.

Practical Dietary Adjustments:

- Limit Red and Processed Meats: Reduce intake of red meats and processed meats. Opt for leaner protein sources, such as poultry, fish, and plant-based proteins like beans and legumes.
- Incorporate Plant-Based Proteins: Explore plant-based protein options such as tofu, tempeh, and lentils. These foods provide essential nutrients without the inflammatory effects associated with red and processed meats.

4. Refined Carbohydrates

Concept and Impact:

Refined carbohydrates, found in white bread, pastries, and other processed grain products, can contribute to inflammation and chronic pain. These carbohydrates are quickly broken down into glucose, leading to spikes in blood sugar levels.

- Blood Sugar Spikes: Refined carbohydrates can cause rapid increases in blood glucose, leading to insulin resistance and inflammation. This contributes to a cycle of increased pain and discomfort.
- Nutrient Deficiency: Foods made from refined carbohydrates often lack essential nutrients and fiber, which are important for overall health and managing inflammation.

Practical Dietary Adjustments:

- Choose Whole Grains: Replace refined carbohydrates with whole grains, such as brown rice, quinoa, and whole wheat products. These options provide more fiber and nutrients that help manage inflammation.
- Read Nutrition Labels: Pay attention to ingredient lists and choose products labeled as "whole grain" or "100% whole wheat" to ensure that you are consuming more nutrient-dense options.

5. Artificial Additives and Preservatives

Concept and Impact:

Artificial additives and preservatives used in processed foods can contribute to inflammation and exacerbate chronic pain. These substances may include artificial sweeteners, colors, flavors, and preservatives.

- Inflammatory Effects: Some artificial additives and preservatives have been linked to increased inflammation and adverse health effects. For example, certain artificial colors and flavors may trigger inflammatory responses in sensitive individuals.
- Health Implications: Long-term consumption of foods containing artificial additives can affect gut health, immune function, and overall well-being, potentially worsening chronic pain conditions.

Practical Dietary Adjustments:

- Minimize Processed Foods: Avoid foods with a long list of artificial ingredients and preservatives. Focus on fresh, whole foods with minimal processing to reduce exposure to harmful additives.
- Read Labels Carefully: Check nutrition labels for artificial additives and choose products with simple, natural ingredients. Opt for organic or minimally processed options when possible.

CREATING A BALANCED DIET PLAN

Creating a balanced diet plan is essential for managing chronic pain and supporting overall health. A well-structured diet plan should address nutritional needs, incorporate anti-inflammatory foods, and avoid foods that can exacerbate pain. This section provides a comprehensive guide to developing a balanced diet plan tailored to individual needs, including practical tips, meal planning strategies, and sample meal ideas.

1. Understanding Nutritional Needs

Concept and Importance:

A balanced diet provides the body with essential nutrients required for optimal function and health. Understanding nutritional needs involves recognizing the role of macronutrients (carbohydrates, proteins, and fats) and micronutrients (vitamins and minerals) in managing chronic pain and supporting overall well-being.

- Macronutrients: Carbohydrates provide energy, proteins are vital for tissue repair and immune function, and fats support cell health and hormone production. Balancing these macronutrients is crucial for maintaining energy levels and managing inflammation.
- Micronutrients: Vitamins and minerals play roles in reducing inflammation and supporting various bodily functions. For instance, vitamin D and calcium are important for bone health, while antioxidants like vitamin C and E help combat oxidative stress.

Practical Dietary Adjustments:

- Assess Individual Needs: Consult with a healthcare professional or dietitian to assess your specific nutritional needs based on factors such as age, sex, activity level, and health conditions.
- Incorporate Nutrient-Dense Foods: Focus on incorporating nutrient-dense foods into your diet, including a variety of fruits, vegetables, whole grains, lean proteins, and healthy fats.

2. Designing a Meal Plan

Concept and Importance:

Designing a meal plan helps ensure that you meet your nutritional needs while managing chronic pain. A well-balanced meal plan includes a variety of foods, portion control, and timing of meals to optimize nutrient intake and maintain steady energy levels.

- Meal Frequency and Timing: Eating smaller, frequent meals can help maintain energy levels and manage blood sugar. Include balanced meals and snacks throughout the day to avoid spikes and crashes in energy.
- Portion Control: Managing portion sizes is important for maintaining a healthy weight and avoiding overeating. Use tools like measuring cups or a food scale to help with portion control.

Practical Dietary Adjustments:

- Create a Weekly Menu: Plan meals and snacks for the week, including breakfast, lunch, dinner, and snacks. Ensure that each meal includes a balance of macronutrients and a variety of colorful fruits and vegetables.
- Prepare in Advance: Prepare meals in advance to save time and ensure you have healthy options readily available. Consider batch cooking and storing meals in portion-sized containers.

3. Balancing Macronutrients

Concept and Importance:

Balancing macronutrients is key to managing chronic pain and supporting overall health. Each macronutrient plays a unique role in the body, and achieving the right balance can help reduce inflammation and maintain energy levels.

- Carbohydrates: Choose complex carbohydrates such as whole grains, legumes, and vegetables. These provide sustained energy and support digestive health. Limit simple carbohydrates like sugary snacks and refined grains.
- Proteins: Include a variety of protein sources, such as lean meats, fish, beans, and tofu. Protein is essential for muscle repair, immune function, and overall health.
- Fats: Focus on healthy fats, such as those found in avocados, nuts, seeds, and fatty fish. These fats have anti-inflammatory properties and support overall health.

Practical Dietary Adjustments:
- Create Balanced Meals: Ensure each meal includes a source of carbohydrates, proteins, and healthy fats. For example, a meal might include grilled chicken (protein), quinoa (carbohydrate), and avocado (fat).
- Monitor Macronutrient Ratios: Use a food diary or app to track macronutrient intake and adjust portions as needed to achieve a balanced diet.

4. Incorporating Anti-Inflammatory Foods

Concept and Importance:

Incorporating anti-inflammatory foods into your diet can help manage chronic pain and reduce inflammation. These foods contain compounds that combat inflammation and support overall health.

- Fruits and Vegetables: Include a variety of colorful fruits and vegetables rich in antioxidants, vitamins, and minerals. Aim for at least five servings of fruits and vegetables per day.
- Healthy Fats: Incorporate sources of omega-3 fatty acids, such as fatty fish, nuts, and seeds. These fats help reduce inflammation and support joint health.
- Whole Grains: Choose whole grains over refined grains to provide fiber and essential nutrients. Whole grains help regulate blood sugar levels and reduce inflammation.

Practical Dietary Adjustments:

- Create an Anti-Inflammatory Shopping List: Include foods such as berries, leafy greens, fatty fish, nuts, and whole grains in your shopping list. Avoid foods that are high in refined sugars, unhealthy fats, and artificial additives.
- Incorporate Anti-Inflammatory Recipes: Explore recipes that feature anti-inflammatory ingredients. For example, prepare a salad with mixed greens, berries, and nuts, or bake salmon with a turmeric and ginger marinade.

5. Avoiding Pro-Inflammatory Foods

Concept and Importance:

Avoiding pro-inflammatory foods is crucial for managing chronic pain and reducing inflammation.

Certain foods can trigger or worsen inflammation, leading to increased pain and discomfort.

- Refined Sugars and Processed Foods: Limit the intake of foods high in refined sugars, trans fats, and processed additives. These foods can contribute to systemic inflammation and worsen chronic pain conditions.
- Red and Processed Meats: Reduce consumption of red and processed meats, which are high in saturated fats and additives that can exacerbate inflammation.

Practical Dietary Adjustments:

- Read Nutrition Labels: Check labels for added sugars, unhealthy fats, and artificial ingredients. Choose products with minimal processing and fewer additives.
- Opt for Whole Food Alternatives: Replace processed snacks and meals with whole food options, such as fresh fruits, vegetables, and homemade meals.

6. Monitoring and Adjusting Your Plan

Concept and Importance:

Regular monitoring and adjusting your diet plan are essential for ensuring its effectiveness in managing chronic pain and meeting nutritional needs. Flexibility and periodic evaluation can help you make necessary adjustments based on your health and lifestyle changes.

- Track Progress: Use a food diary or app to monitor your diet, note any changes in pain levels, and assess how well your diet plan is working. Tracking progress helps identify patterns and make informed adjustments.
- Consult with Professionals: Regularly consult with a healthcare provider or dietitian to review your diet plan, address any concerns, and make adjustments based on your evolving needs and health goals.

Practical Dietary Adjustments:

- Adjust Based on Feedback: Modify your diet plan based on feedback from your healthcare provider and personal observations. If certain foods exacerbate pain or cause discomfort, consider eliminating or reducing them.
- Stay Informed: Keep up-to-date with the latest research on nutrition and chronic pain management. Incorporate new findings into your diet plan to ensure it remains effective and relevant.

CHAPTER 6

PAIN MANAGEMENT TOOLS AND TECHNIQUES

HEAT AND COLD THERAPY

Heat and cold therapy are fundamental methods used in pain management. These therapies can help alleviate pain, reduce inflammation, and improve function. Understanding when and how to use heat and cold therapy effectively can significantly impact pain relief and recovery. This section delves into the principles behind each therapy, their benefits, applications, and best practices for use.

1. Heat Therapy
Concept and Benefits:
Heat therapy involves applying warmth to the body to relieve pain, reduce muscle stiffness, and improve blood circulation. It is commonly used for chronic pain conditions and muscle tension.

- Mechanism of Action: Heat therapy works by dilating blood vessels, which increases blood flow to the affected area. This improved circulation helps deliver more oxygen and nutrients while removing metabolic waste products, which can reduce muscle tension and stiffness.

- Benefits: Heat therapy can help soothe sore muscles, alleviate joint pain, and increase flexibility. It is particularly effective for conditions such as arthritis, menstrual cramps, and chronic back pain.

Types of Heat Therapy:

- Dry Heat: Uses materials such as heating pads or hot water bottles. Dry heat is convenient and can be applied directly to the skin, but it is important to use a barrier (such as a towel) to prevent burns.
- Moist Heat: Includes methods such as warm, damp towels, or steam packs. Moist heat can penetrate deeper into the tissues and may be more effective for relieving stiffness and pain.

Application Tips:

- Duration: Apply heat therapy for 15-20 minutes at a time, allowing the skin to return to its normal temperature before reapplying. Excessive heat can cause burns or worsen inflammation.
- Temperature: Ensure that the heat source is warm, not hot, to avoid burns. Test the temperature on a small area of skin before applying it to the affected area.

2. Cold Therapy

Concept and Benefits:

Cold therapy, or cryotherapy, involves applying cold to the body to reduce inflammation, numb pain, and decrease swelling. It is commonly used for acute injuries and inflammatory conditions.

- Mechanism of Action: Cold therapy works by constricting blood vessels, which reduces blood flow and limits the inflammatory response. This helps numb the affected area and can minimize swelling and pain.
- Benefits: Cold therapy is effective for acute injuries such as sprains, strains, and bruises. It can also help reduce inflammation and manage pain in conditions like arthritis and tendonitis.

Types of Cold Therapy:

- Ice Packs: Commonly used for acute injuries, ice packs can be made from ice cubes wrapped in a cloth or purchased as gel packs. They are effective for reducing swelling and numbing pain.
- Cold Compresses: These are pre-made cold packs or wraps that can be stored in the freezer. Cold compresses are convenient and can be applied directly to the skin.

Application Tips:

- Duration: Apply cold therapy for 10-15 minutes at a time, with a break of at least 1 hour between applications. Prolonged exposure to cold can cause frostbite or damage to the skin.

- Temperature: Use a barrier such as a towel or cloth between the ice pack and the skin to prevent frostbite. Ensure that the cold source is not directly applied to the skin for extended periods.

3. Combining Heat and Cold Therapy

Concept and Benefits:

In some cases, alternating between heat and cold therapy can provide enhanced relief for certain types of pain or conditions. This approach can help address both acute inflammation and chronic muscle tension.

- Alternating Therapy: Alternating between heat and cold can help reduce muscle spasms, improve blood flow, and alleviate pain. This method is often referred to as contrast therapy.
- Benefits: Combining heat and cold therapy can provide a balanced approach to pain management, addressing both the inflammatory and muscle tension aspects of chronic pain.

Application Tips:

- Cycle Duration: Alternate between heat and cold therapy every 15-20 minutes. For example, apply heat for 15 minutes, followed by cold therapy for 15 minutes, and repeat as needed.
- Monitor Responses: Pay attention to how your body responds to each therapy. Adjust the

duration and frequency of application based on your comfort and pain relief.

4. Precautions and Considerations

Concept and Importance:

While heat and cold therapy can be highly effective, it is important to use these methods safely and appropriately. Certain conditions and precautions should be considered to avoid adverse effects.

- Skin Sensitivity: Individuals with sensitive skin, poor circulation, or conditions such as diabetes should exercise caution when using heat and cold therapy. Consult with a healthcare provider before starting these therapies.

- Medical Conditions: Avoid heat therapy if you have acute inflammation or swelling, as heat can worsen these conditions. Similarly, avoid cold therapy if you have poor circulation or certain skin conditions.

Practical Considerations:

- Consult a Professional: Always consult with a healthcare provider to determine the most appropriate therapy for your specific condition and to receive personalized recommendations.

- Monitor Reactions: Pay close attention to your body's response to heat and cold therapy. Discontinue use if you experience increased pain, discomfort, or adverse reactions.

MASSAGE AND MANUAL THERAPY

Massage and manual therapy are therapeutic techniques used to alleviate pain, enhance physical function, and promote overall well-being. These approaches involve the use of hands-on techniques to manipulate the body's soft tissues, such as muscles, tendons, and ligaments. They can be particularly effective for managing chronic pain, reducing muscle tension, and improving circulation. This section provides an in-depth exploration of massage and manual therapy, including their types, benefits, techniques, and considerations for their use.

1. Understanding Massage Therapy

Concept and Benefits:

Massage therapy involves applying varying degrees of pressure and manipulation to the body's soft tissues to relieve pain, reduce stress, and promote relaxation. It is commonly used for its therapeutic benefits in treating chronic pain conditions and enhancing overall health.

- Mechanism of Action: Massage therapy works by stimulating blood flow, relaxing muscle tissues, and breaking down adhesions or scar tissue. This can lead to improved circulation, reduced muscle tension, and relief from pain.
- Benefits: Regular massage therapy can help reduce chronic pain, improve range of motion, alleviate stress and anxiety, and enhance overall

physical function. It is often used in conjunction with other pain management strategies.

Types of Massage Therapy:

- Swedish Massage: This technique uses long, flowing strokes, kneading, and circular movements to relax muscles and improve circulation. It is beneficial for general relaxation and easing muscle tension.

- Deep Tissue Massage: This method focuses on the deeper layers of muscle and connective tissue, using slow, deep strokes to address chronic muscle pain and stiffness. It is effective for targeting specific areas of discomfort.

- Trigger Point Therapy: This technique involves applying pressure to specific points in the muscles to relieve areas of intense pain and tightness. It helps to release muscle knots and improve function.

Application Tips:

- Frequency: The frequency of massage therapy sessions can vary based on individual needs and conditions. Regular sessions may be beneficial for chronic pain management, while occasional sessions can provide relief for acute issues.

- Choosing a Therapist: Select a licensed and experienced massage therapist who specializes in your specific condition or pain management needs. Discuss your goals and any concerns before starting therapy.

2. Understanding Manual Therapy

Concept and Benefits:

Manual therapy encompasses a range of hands-on techniques designed to improve musculoskeletal function, reduce pain, and enhance mobility. It includes various approaches that focus on the manipulation and mobilization of joints and soft tissues.

- Mechanism of Action: Manual therapy techniques work by applying controlled force to joints and tissues, aiming to restore normal movement patterns, reduce stiffness, and alleviate pain. Techniques may involve stretching, joint mobilization, and manipulation.
- Benefits: Manual therapy can help improve joint range of motion, reduce pain and muscle tension, enhance tissue healing, and promote overall functional improvement. It is often used as part of a comprehensive treatment plan.

Types of Manual Therapy:

- Joint Mobilization: This technique involves applying gentle, controlled movements to a joint to improve its range of motion and reduce stiffness. It is effective for addressing joint dysfunction and pain.
- Joint Manipulation: This approach uses a quick, controlled force to adjust the position of a joint

and restore normal function. It is often used to relieve pain and improve joint mobility.

- Soft Tissue Mobilization: This technique focuses on manipulating the soft tissues, such as muscles, tendons, and fascia, to reduce pain, improve circulation, and enhance flexibility.

Application Tips:

- Assessment: Before starting manual therapy, a thorough assessment by a qualified practitioner is essential to identify specific issues and develop an appropriate treatment plan.
- Integration: Manual therapy can be integrated with other therapeutic approaches, such as exercise and stretching, to enhance overall effectiveness and support long-term pain management.

3. Benefits of Combining Massage and Manual Therapy

Concept and Benefits:

Combining massage and manual therapy can offer a holistic approach to pain management and physical rehabilitation. Each therapy complements the other, addressing different aspects of pain and dysfunction.

- Enhanced Pain Relief: The combination of massage and manual therapy can provide comprehensive pain relief by targeting both soft tissue and joint issues. This integrated approach can lead to more effective and lasting results.

- Improved Function: By addressing muscle tension, joint restrictions, and soft tissue dysfunction, the combination of therapies can enhance overall physical function and mobility.

Practical Considerations:

- Personalized Treatment Plan: Work with a healthcare provider or therapist to develop a personalized treatment plan that incorporates both massage and manual therapy based on your specific needs and goals.
- Monitor Progress: Regularly assess your progress and adjust the therapy plan as needed. Communicate with your therapist about any changes in pain, function, or comfort levels.

4. Safety and Precautions

Concept and Importance:

While massage and manual therapy can be highly beneficial, it is important to use these techniques safely and consider individual health conditions and needs. Certain precautions should be taken to ensure safe and effective treatment.

- Medical Conditions: Inform your therapist of any pre-existing medical conditions, injuries, or health concerns that may affect your ability to receive massage or manual therapy. Certain conditions may require modifications or contraindications.

- Proper Technique: Ensure that your therapist uses proper techniques and maintains appropriate pressure to avoid injury or discomfort. Always communicate openly about any pain or discomfort experienced during the session.

Practical Considerations:

- Consult a Professional: Seek guidance from a qualified healthcare provider or therapist to determine if massage and manual therapy are appropriate for your specific condition and to receive personalized recommendations.
- Follow Recommendations: Adhere to any recommendations or guidelines provided by your therapist, including frequency of sessions, self-care practices, and complementary therapies.

ACUPUNCTURE AND ALTERNATIVE TREATMENTS

Acupuncture and alternative treatments encompass a range of therapies used to manage chronic pain and improve overall health. These approaches often draw from traditional and complementary medicine practices, offering additional options for individuals seeking relief from persistent pain. This section explores the principles, benefits, techniques, and considerations of acupuncture and other alternative treatments.

1. Acupuncture

Concept and Benefits:

Acupuncture is a traditional Chinese medicine practice that involves inserting thin needles into specific points on the body, known as acupuncture points, to stimulate the body's natural healing processes and restore balance. It is widely used to alleviate pain and treat various health conditions.

- Mechanism of Action: Acupuncture is based on the concept of Qi (pronounced "chee"), which is believed to flow through pathways in the body called meridians. By stimulating specific acupuncture points, practitioners aim to regulate the flow of Qi, improve energy balance, and promote healing.
- Benefits: Acupuncture can help reduce chronic pain, enhance pain management, improve circulation, and support overall well-being. It is often used for conditions such as back pain, arthritis, headaches, and fibromyalgia.

Types of Acupuncture:

- Traditional Chinese Acupuncture: This approach follows traditional Chinese medicine principles, using specific points along meridians to balance Qi and treat a range of health issues.
- Electro-Acupuncture: Involves applying a small electric current to the acupuncture needles to

enhance the therapeutic effects. It is often used for pain relief and muscle stimulation.

- Auricular Acupuncture: Focuses on specific points on the ear, which are believed to correspond to different parts of the body. It is used to address various health concerns, including pain and addiction.

Application Tips:

- Frequency: The frequency of acupuncture sessions varies based on individual needs and conditions. Initial treatments may be more frequent, with a gradual reduction in frequency as symptoms improve.
- Choosing a Practitioner: Select a licensed and experienced acupuncturist who adheres to recognized standards and practices. Discuss your health goals and any concerns before starting treatment.

2. Alternative Treatments

Concept and Benefits:

Alternative treatments include a variety of non-conventional therapies that can complement traditional medical approaches. These treatments often focus on holistic care and addressing the root causes of pain.

Types of Alternative Treatments:

- Chiropractic Care: Involves the manual adjustment of the spine and other joints to improve alignment, reduce pain, and enhance function. Chiropractors use techniques such as spinal manipulation to address musculoskeletal issues.

- **Benefits**: Chiropractic care can help relieve back pain, neck pain, and headaches. It may also improve joint mobility and reduce muscle tension.

- **Application Tips:** Consult with a licensed chiropractor to develop a personalized treatment plan. Chiropractic adjustments should be performed by a qualified professional to ensure safety and effectiveness.

- Osteopathic Manipulative Treatment (OMT): Utilizes hands-on techniques to diagnose, treat, and prevent conditions related to the bones, muscles, and joints. OMT is performed by osteopathic physicians (DOs) who are trained in both conventional and osteopathic medicine.

- **Benefits**: OMT can help alleviate pain, improve function, and enhance overall health. It is often used for conditions such as musculoskeletal pain, headaches, and joint issues.

- **Application Tips:** Work with a licensed DO who specializes in OMT to receive tailored care based on your specific needs and health goals.

- Herbal Medicine: Involves using plant-based remedies to support health and alleviate symptoms. Herbal medicine can include teas, supplements, and tinctures made from herbs with known therapeutic properties.

- **Benefits**: Herbal remedies can provide relief from various conditions, including pain, inflammation, and digestive issues. They are often used in combination with other treatments for enhanced effects.

- **Application Tips:** Consult with a qualified herbalist or healthcare provider to select appropriate herbs and ensure safe usage. Be aware of potential interactions with other medications.

- Homeopathy: A system of medicine based on the principle of "like cures like," where highly diluted substances are used to stimulate the body's healing response. Homeopathic remedies are tailored to individual symptoms and overall health.

- **Benefits:** Homeopathy can address a wide range of conditions, including chronic pain, stress, and allergies. It aims to support the body's natural healing processes.

- **Application Tips**: Seek guidance from a licensed homeopath or healthcare provider to select appropriate remedies and ensure they align with your health needs.

3. Integrating Acupuncture and Alternative Treatments
Concept and Benefits:
Combining acupuncture and alternative treatments with conventional medical approaches can provide a comprehensive pain management strategy. These therapies can complement traditional treatments, enhance overall effectiveness, and address various aspects of chronic pain.

- Holistic Approach: Integrating these therapies allows for a more holistic approach to pain management, addressing physical, emotional, and energetic aspects of health.
- Personalized Care: Combining therapies enables a tailored treatment plan that aligns with individual needs and preferences, providing a more personalized approach to pain management.

Practical Considerations:

- Consult with Professionals: Work with healthcare providers who are knowledgeable about both conventional and alternative treatments to develop a well-rounded treatment plan.
- Monitor Progress: Regularly assess the effectiveness of combined therapies and adjust the treatment plan as needed. Communicate openly with your healthcare providers about any changes or concerns.

4. Safety and Precautions

Concept and Importance:

While acupuncture and alternative treatments can offer significant benefits, it is important to use them safely and consider individual health conditions. Certain precautions should be taken to ensure effective and safe treatment.

- Medical Conditions: Inform your practitioners of any pre-existing medical conditions, medications, or health concerns that may affect the use of alternative treatments. Some therapies may require modifications or contraindications.
- Qualified Practitioners: Ensure that you receive treatments from licensed and qualified professionals who adhere to recognized standards and practices. This helps ensure safety and effectiveness.

Practical Considerations:

- Consult a Professional: Seek guidance from healthcare providers to determine if acupuncture and alternative treatments are appropriate for your specific condition and to receive personalized recommendations.
- Evaluate Responses: Pay close attention to your body's response to each therapy. Adjust the frequency, type, or combination of treatments based on your comfort and progress.

USING ASSISTIVE DEVICES

Assistive devices play a crucial role in managing chronic pain and improving daily function for individuals with various health conditions. These tools can help alleviate discomfort, enhance mobility, and support independence. This section explores different types of assistive devices, their benefits, usage tips, and considerations for integrating them into a comprehensive pain management plan.

1. Types of Assistive Devices

Concept and Benefits:

Assistive devices are designed to support individuals in performing daily activities more comfortably and effectively. They range from simple tools to complex machines, each serving specific purposes to address different aspects of pain and disability.

Categories of Assistive Devices:

- Mobility Aids: These devices assist with movement and stability, making it easier to navigate different environments.
    - Canes and Walking Sticks: Provide support and balance, reducing the risk of falls and alleviating pressure on affected joints.
    - Walkers and Rollators: Offer additional support and stability for individuals who require assistance with walking. Rollators

come with wheels and may include seats for resting.

  o Wheelchairs and Power Chairs: Aid individuals with severe mobility impairments by providing means of transportation and reducing the physical strain of walking.

- Ergonomic Tools: Designed to reduce strain and improve comfort during daily activities, especially for individuals with musculoskeletal pain.

  o Ergonomic Chairs: Support proper posture and reduce back pain by providing adjustable features such as lumbar support, seat height, and armrests.

  o Adaptive Workstations: Include adjustable desks, computer stands, and ergonomic keyboards that help minimize strain during work or computer use.

  o Reacher Graspers: Help individuals with limited mobility reach and grasp objects without bending or stretching.

- Pain Relief Devices: These tools provide direct relief from pain through various methods.

  o TENS Units (Transcutaneous Electrical Nerve Stimulation): Deliver electrical impulses to nerves through electrodes, helping to reduce pain by stimulating the release of endorphins and blocking pain signals.

- ○ Heating Pads and Cold Packs: Offer thermal therapy to alleviate pain and reduce inflammation. Heating pads relax muscles and improve blood flow, while cold packs reduce swelling and numb pain.
- ○ Massage Devices: Include handheld massagers and percussion devices that provide targeted relief by soothing sore muscles and improving circulation.

- Supportive Braces and Orthotics: Provide additional support and stabilization to affected areas, reducing pain and improving function.
  - ○ Joint Braces: Help stabilize and support injured or weak joints, such as knee or wrist braces. They can prevent excessive movement and alleviate discomfort.
  - ○ Orthotic Insoles: Provide cushioning and support to the feet, improving alignment and reducing strain on the lower body.

2. Benefits of Using Assistive Devices

Concept and Benefits:

Using assistive devices can offer numerous benefits for individuals managing chronic pain, enhancing their quality of life and daily functioning.

- Pain Relief: Devices such as TENS units and heating pads provide direct pain relief by addressing the source of discomfort and reducing inflammation.
- Improved Mobility: Mobility aids and ergonomic tools help individuals move more easily and comfortably, reducing physical strain and enhancing overall mobility.
- Enhanced Independence: Assistive devices empower individuals to perform daily activities with greater ease, promoting independence and self-sufficiency.
- Increased Comfort: Ergonomic tools and supportive devices improve comfort during work and leisure activities, reducing strain and preventing exacerbation of pain.

3. Choosing and Using Assistive Devices

Concept and Considerations:

Selecting and using the right assistive devices requires careful consideration of individual needs, preferences, and specific health conditions. Here are key factors to consider:

- Assessment: Consult with a healthcare professional, such as an occupational therapist or physical therapist, to assess your specific needs and determine the most suitable assistive devices.
- Personal Fit: Ensure that devices are appropriately sized and adjusted to fit your body

and activity level. For example, ergonomic chairs and braces should be tailored to your measurements and comfort.

- Ease of Use: Choose devices that are easy to use and incorporate into your daily routine. Consider factors such as weight, ease of adjustment, and user-friendliness.
- Cost and Insurance: Evaluate the cost of assistive devices and check if they are covered by insurance or available through health programs. Some devices may require a prescription or approval for insurance reimbursement.

4. Integrating Assistive Devices into Your Routine

Concept and Benefits:

Effectively integrating assistive devices into your daily routine can enhance their benefits and improve overall pain management.

- Routine Use: Incorporate devices into your daily activities as recommended by your healthcare provider. For example, use ergonomic tools at work and mobility aids during physical activities.
- Regular Maintenance: Ensure that devices are properly maintained and kept in good working condition. Regularly inspect and clean devices, and replace any worn or damaged components.
- Monitoring Effectiveness: Regularly assess the effectiveness of assistive devices and make adjustments as needed. Communicate with your

healthcare provider about any changes in pain levels or functionality.

5. Safety and Precautions

Concept and Importance:

Using assistive devices safely is crucial to prevent injury and ensure effective pain management. Follow these precautions to maximize the benefits and minimize risks:

- Proper Usage: Follow the manufacturer's instructions and recommendations for each device. Incorrect use may lead to discomfort or exacerbate existing issues.
- Consultation: Consult with a healthcare professional before using new assistive devices, especially if you have specific health conditions or concerns.
- Monitor for Issues: Pay attention to any adverse effects or discomfort while using assistive devices. If you experience any issues, seek guidance from a healthcare provider for potential adjustments or alternatives.

CHAPTER 7

UNDERSTANDING THE EMOTIONAL IMPACT

Chronic pain often exerts a significant emotional toll on individuals, affecting their mental well-being and overall quality of life. This emotional impact can manifest in various ways, influencing not only how individuals perceive and cope with their pain but also their interactions with others and their daily functioning. Understanding these emotional aspects is crucial for providing comprehensive support and developing effective strategies for managing chronic pain.

1. Emotional Responses to Chronic Pain

Concept and Types of Emotional Responses:

The persistent nature of chronic pain can lead to a range of emotional responses, each affecting individuals differently. Recognizing and addressing these responses is essential for holistic pain management.

- Frustration and Anger: Chronic pain can cause frustration and anger due to the constant discomfort and limitations it imposes. Individuals may feel helpless or resentful about their inability to engage in activities they once enjoyed or to achieve their personal goals.

- Anxiety and Worry: Persistent pain often leads to anxiety about the future, including concerns about worsening symptoms, the impact on one's ability to work, and the potential for reduced independence. This anxiety can exacerbate the perception of pain and contribute to a cycle of stress and discomfort.

- Depression: Chronic pain is closely linked with depression, characterized by feelings of sadness, hopelessness, and a lack of interest in daily activities. The ongoing struggle with pain can lead to emotional withdrawal, decreased motivation, and a negative outlook on life.

- Isolation and Loneliness: The limitations imposed by chronic pain can result in social withdrawal and isolation. Individuals may avoid social interactions or activities due to pain, leading to feelings of loneliness and a reduced sense of connection with others.

2. The Interaction Between Pain and Emotions

Concept and Implications:

Emotions and pain are interconnected, influencing each other in complex ways. Understanding this interaction is vital for addressing both physical and emotional aspects of chronic pain.

- Pain Amplification: Emotional distress can amplify the perception of pain. Stress, anxiety, and depression can heighten pain sensitivity and contribute to a more intense experience of discomfort.

- Pain Management Challenges: Emotional struggles can complicate pain management efforts. For example, individuals experiencing depression may have difficulty adhering to treatment plans or engaging in self-care practices, impacting their overall pain management.
- Feedback Loop: The interplay between pain and emotions creates a feedback loop, where emotional distress exacerbates pain, and pain intensifies emotional suffering. Addressing both aspects simultaneously is essential for effective pain management.

3. Strategies for Managing Emotional Impact

Concept and Approaches:

Developing strategies to manage the emotional impact of chronic pain is crucial for improving overall well-being and enhancing quality of life. Several approaches can help individuals cope with the emotional challenges associated with chronic pain.

- Cognitive-Behavioral Therapy (CBT): CBT is a widely used therapeutic approach that helps individuals identify and change negative thought patterns and behaviors related to pain. By addressing cognitive distortions and promoting healthier coping strategies, CBT can alleviate emotional distress and improve pain management.

- Mindfulness and Relaxation Techniques: Mindfulness practices, such as meditation and deep breathing exercises, can help individuals manage stress and anxiety. These techniques promote relaxation, enhance self-awareness, and provide tools for coping with pain.
- Support Groups and Counseling: Engaging in support groups or individual counseling provides a platform for sharing experiences, gaining emotional support, and learning from others facing similar challenges. Professional counseling can offer tailored strategies and emotional support to address individual needs.
- Lifestyle Modifications: Incorporating lifestyle changes, such as regular physical activity, healthy eating, and adequate sleep, can positively impact emotional well-being. These changes contribute to overall health and can help mitigate the emotional effects of chronic pain.

4. The Role of Social Support

Concept and Importance:

Social support plays a crucial role in managing the emotional impact of chronic pain. Having a network of supportive friends, family members, and healthcare professionals can provide significant benefits.

- Emotional Support: Having a supportive network helps individuals feel understood and validated. Emotional support from loved ones can reduce feelings of isolation and provide encouragement and empathy.

- Practical Assistance: Social support can also include practical assistance, such as help with daily tasks, transportation to medical appointments, or support with managing pain-related challenges.

- Open Communication: Maintaining open and honest communication with friends, family, and healthcare providers fosters a supportive environment and helps address emotional concerns. Encouraging dialogue about pain and its impact promotes understanding and collaboration in managing chronic pain.

5. Professional Help and Resources

Concept and Resources:

Accessing professional help and resources is essential for addressing the emotional impact of chronic pain and developing effective coping strategies.

- Mental Health Professionals: Seeking assistance from mental health professionals, such as psychologists, psychiatrists, or therapists, can provide valuable support for managing emotional distress. These professionals can offer therapy, medication management, and coping strategies tailored to individual needs.

- Pain Management Clinics: Specialized pain management clinics often have multidisciplinary teams that include psychologists, counselors, and other professionals who can address the emotional aspects of pain. These clinics provide integrated care to support both physical and emotional well-being.
- Educational Resources: Accessing educational resources, such as books, online courses, and workshops, can provide information and tools for managing the emotional impact of chronic pain. These resources offer practical strategies and insights into coping with emotional challenges.

COPING STRATEGIES FOR EMOTIONAL WELL-BEING

Managing chronic pain involves not only addressing physical symptoms but also tackling the emotional and psychological challenges that come with it. Effective coping strategies are crucial for maintaining emotional well-being and improving overall quality of life. This section delves into various coping strategies designed to help individuals manage the emotional aspects of chronic pain, offering practical approaches and techniques to foster resilience and mental health.

1. Cognitive-Behavioral Strategies

Concept and Techniques:

Cognitive-behavioral strategies are effective for altering negative thought patterns and behaviors related to chronic pain. These techniques focus on changing how individuals think about and respond to their pain, thereby improving emotional well-being.

- Cognitive Restructuring: This technique involves identifying and challenging negative or distorted thoughts about pain. By replacing these thoughts with more balanced and realistic perspectives, individuals can reduce feelings of helplessness and improve their coping abilities. For example, shifting from "I can never do anything because of my pain" to "I can still find enjoyable activities that accommodate my pain" can lead to a more positive outlook.
- Behavioral Activation: Encouraging engagement in meaningful activities despite pain can help combat feelings of depression and inactivity. Setting small, achievable goals and gradually increasing activity levels can boost mood and enhance a sense of accomplishment.
- Problem-Solving Skills: Developing problem-solving skills helps individuals address

practical challenges associated with chronic pain. This involves identifying problems, brainstorming solutions, and implementing strategies to overcome obstacles, thus reducing stress and frustration.

2. Mindfulness and Relaxation Techniques
Concept and Benefits:

Mindfulness and relaxation techniques help individuals manage stress, anxiety, and emotional distress by promoting relaxation and present-moment awareness. These practices can improve emotional regulation and enhance coping with chronic pain.

- Mindfulness Meditation: Mindfulness meditation involves focusing attention on the present moment without judgment. Regular practice can help individuals observe their pain and emotions with greater detachment, reducing the intensity of their emotional responses. Techniques such as body scans and mindful breathing can increase awareness and acceptance of pain.
- Deep Breathing Exercises: Deep breathing exercises help activate the body's relaxation response, reducing stress and anxiety. Techniques such as diaphragmatic breathing and paced breathing involve slow, deep breaths that can

calm the nervous system and decrease pain perception.

- Progressive Muscle Relaxation (PMR): PMR involves systematically tensing and then relaxing different muscle groups to alleviate physical and emotional tension. By focusing on the contrast between tension and relaxation, individuals can experience reduced muscle tightness and improved overall relaxation.

3. Emotional Expression and Processing

Concept and Methods:

Expressing and processing emotions are crucial for managing the emotional impact of chronic pain. Allowing oneself to acknowledge and work through emotions can lead to greater emotional resilience and well-being.

- Journaling: Keeping a journal provides a safe space for individuals to express their thoughts and feelings related to chronic pain. Writing about pain experiences, emotions, and coping strategies can help process and release pent-up emotions, leading to greater self-awareness and emotional clarity.
- Creative Outlets: Engaging in creative activities such as painting, drawing, or crafting can serve as an emotional outlet and provide a sense of accomplishment. Creative expression allows

individuals to channel their emotions in a constructive way and can enhance mood and reduce stress.

- Therapeutic Expression: Participating in therapy, such as art therapy or music therapy, offers additional avenues for emotional expression and processing. These therapies can help individuals explore and express their emotions through creative means, promoting emotional healing and resilience.

4. Building and Maintaining Social Support

Concept and Importance:

Social support is vital for emotional well-being, providing individuals with a sense of connection, understanding, and encouragement. Building and maintaining strong social relationships can significantly impact emotional health and coping with chronic pain.

- Connecting with Support Networks: Engaging with family, friends, and support groups helps individuals share their experiences and receive emotional support. Social connections provide empathy, validation, and practical assistance, reducing feelings of isolation and loneliness.
- Participating in Support Groups: Support groups for chronic pain or related conditions offer a platform for individuals to connect with others facing similar challenges. These groups provide

mutual support, shared experiences, and valuable coping strategies.

- Communicating Needs and Boundaries: Open communication with loved ones about pain, needs, and limitations is essential for building supportive relationships. Expressing needs and setting boundaries helps others understand how to offer support effectively and reduces misunderstandings.

5. Professional Help and Therapy

Concept and Benefits:

Seeking professional help and therapy can provide targeted support for managing the emotional aspects of chronic pain. Various therapeutic approaches offer valuable tools and strategies for improving emotional well-being.

- Cognitive-Behavioral Therapy (CBT): CBT focuses on modifying negative thought patterns and behaviors associated with chronic pain. By addressing cognitive distortions and teaching coping skills, CBT helps individuals develop healthier perspectives and coping strategies.
- Acceptance and Commitment Therapy (ACT): ACT encourages individuals to accept pain and focus on living a meaningful life despite its presence. By promoting psychological flexibility and commitment to personal values, ACT helps

individuals improve emotional resilience and overall well-being.

- Counseling and Psychotherapy: Individual counseling and psychotherapy provide a supportive space to explore emotional challenges, develop coping skills, and work through psychological barriers. Therapists offer personalized strategies and guidance to address specific emotional concerns.

6. Lifestyle and Self-Care Practices

Concept and Strategies:

Incorporating lifestyle and self-care practices into daily routines can enhance emotional well-being and support overall health. These practices contribute to a balanced approach to managing chronic pain.

- Regular Physical Activity: Engaging in regular exercise can improve mood, reduce stress, and enhance overall well-being. Physical activity stimulates the release of endorphins, which can elevate mood and alleviate pain.

- Healthy Eating: A balanced diet supports overall health and can positively impact emotional well-being. Nutrient-rich foods, including fruits, vegetables, and whole grains, contribute to improved mood and energy levels.

- Adequate Sleep: Prioritizing good sleep hygiene and ensuring adequate rest are crucial for emotional resilience. Quality sleep supports mental health and helps manage stress, reducing the emotional impact of chronic pain.

SEEKING PROFESSIONAL SUPPORT

Seeking professional support is a crucial aspect of managing the emotional and psychological challenges associated with chronic pain. Professional help provides individuals with specialized knowledge, tools, and strategies to address both the physical and emotional dimensions of their condition. This section explores the various types of professional support available, how to access these resources, and the benefits they offer in managing chronic pain.

1. Types of Professional Support
Concept and Categories:
Professional support encompasses a range of services and specialties designed to address different aspects of chronic pain management. Each type of professional provides unique insights and interventions that can enhance overall well-being.

- Primary Care Physicians (PCPs): PCPs play a central role in managing chronic pain by overseeing overall health and coordinating care. They can prescribe medications, refer patients to specialists, and provide guidance on managing pain-related conditions. PCPs often serve as the first point of contact and can help develop a comprehensive treatment plan.

- Pain Specialists: Pain specialists, including anesthesiologists and pain management physicians, focus on diagnosing and treating complex pain conditions. They may employ advanced techniques such as nerve blocks, injections, and pain management procedures to address specific pain sources. Pain specialists often work in multidisciplinary settings, collaborating with other healthcare providers to create individualized treatment plans.

- Rheumatologists: Rheumatologists specialize in diagnosing and treating inflammatory and autoimmune disorders that cause chronic pain, such as rheumatoid arthritis and lupus. They provide expertise in managing complex conditions with a focus on reducing inflammation and improving joint function.

- Neurologists: Neurologists address chronic pain conditions related to the nervous system, such as neuropathic pain and migraines. They conduct thorough evaluations to identify neurological causes of pain and recommend appropriate treatments and interventions.

- Psychologists and Psychiatrists: Mental health professionals play a vital role in addressing the psychological and emotional aspects of chronic pain. Psychologists provide therapy, such as cognitive-behavioral therapy (CBT) and acceptance and commitment therapy (ACT), to help individuals manage emotional distress and develop coping skills. Psychiatrists can prescribe medications for conditions like depression and anxiety that may accompany chronic pain.

- Physical Therapists: Physical therapists (PTs) help individuals improve physical function and manage pain through targeted exercise, manual therapy, and education. They design personalized exercise programs to enhance mobility, strength, and flexibility while addressing pain-related limitations.

- Occupational Therapists: Occupational therapists focus on helping individuals adapt to daily activities and improve their quality of life. They provide strategies for managing pain while performing daily tasks, recommend adaptive equipment, and offer training in techniques to minimize pain and enhance independence.

2. How to Access Professional Support

Concept and Steps:

Accessing professional support involves several steps to ensure that individuals receive the appropriate care and services needed for managing chronic pain effectively.

- Consulting with Primary Care Providers: Starting with a primary care provider is often the first step in accessing professional support. PCPs can assess symptoms, provide initial treatment, and refer individuals to specialists if needed. They play a key role in coordinating care and managing overall health.

- Getting Referrals: For specialized care, obtaining referrals from a PCP or other healthcare providers may be necessary. Referrals ensure that individuals are connected with specialists who have expertise in managing specific pain conditions.

- Researching Specialists: Individuals can research pain specialists, rheumatologists, neurologists, and other professionals to find those with experience in treating their specific condition. Online resources, medical directories, and patient reviews can provide valuable information about specialists and their areas of expertise.

- Exploring Insurance Coverage: Understanding insurance coverage is essential for accessing professional support. Checking with insurance providers to determine which services are covered and if referrals are required can help individuals navigate the financial aspects of care.

- Seeking Second Opinions: If there are concerns about a diagnosis or treatment plan, seeking a second opinion from another specialist can provide additional insights and options. Second opinions can help confirm diagnoses and explore alternative treatment approaches.

3. Benefits of Professional Support

Concept and Advantages:

Professional support offers numerous benefits in managing chronic pain, enhancing both physical and emotional well-being.

- Expert Diagnosis and Treatment: Professionals provide accurate diagnoses and develop tailored treatment plans based on their expertise. Their specialized knowledge ensures that individuals receive appropriate and effective interventions for their pain conditions.

- Holistic Approach: Many professionals adopt a holistic approach to pain management, addressing not only physical symptoms but also emotional and psychological aspects. Multidisciplinary care teams work collaboratively to provide comprehensive support and improve overall quality of life.

- Evidence-Based Interventions: Professional support often involves evidence-based interventions and therapies that have been validated through research. This ensures that individuals receive treatments that are proven to be effective and safe.

- Personalized Care: Professionals offer personalized care plans that take into account individual needs, preferences, and goals. Tailoring interventions to each person's unique situation enhances the likelihood of successful outcomes and better management of chronic pain.

- Emotional Support and Guidance: Mental health professionals provide valuable emotional support, helping individuals cope with the psychological challenges of chronic pain. Therapy and counseling can improve emotional resilience, reduce stress, and enhance coping skills.

- Education and Empowerment: Professionals educate individuals about their condition, treatment options, and self-management strategies. This knowledge empowers individuals to actively participate in their care, make informed decisions, and adopt effective self-care practices.

4. Preparing for Professional Appointments

Concept and Tips:

Preparing for appointments with healthcare professionals can help individuals make the most of their time and ensure that all relevant issues are addressed.

- Documenting Symptoms and History: Keeping a detailed record of symptoms, pain patterns, and medical history can provide valuable information for healthcare providers. This documentation helps professionals understand the condition and develop a targeted treatment plan.

- Preparing Questions and Concerns: Prior to appointments, preparing a list of questions and concerns can help individuals address all relevant topics. This ensures that important issues are discussed and that individuals receive clear and comprehensive answers.
- Bringing Support: Bringing a family member or friend to appointments can provide additional support and help remember important information. A support person can also assist in discussing concerns and making decisions about treatment.
- Follow-Up and Communication: Following up on recommendations and maintaining open communication with healthcare providers is crucial for effective management. Regular updates on progress, concerns, and changes in symptoms help professionals adjust treatment plans as needed.

BUILDING A SUPPORT NETWORK

Building a robust support network is an essential strategy for managing chronic pain, as it provides emotional, practical, and social resources that significantly enhance one's quality of life. A well-established support network helps individuals cope with the daily challenges of chronic pain, offers encouragement, and fosters a sense of community and belonging. This section explores the importance of a support network, how to build one, and the benefits it offers.

1. Importance of a Support Network

Concept and Impact:

A support network plays a critical role in managing chronic pain by providing a range of emotional, practical, and informational resources. This network can include family, friends, healthcare professionals, support groups, and online communities. Each component of the support network contributes to a holistic approach to managing chronic pain, addressing various needs and challenges.

- Emotional Support: Having people who understand and empathize with the emotional aspects of chronic pain can reduce feelings of isolation and depression. Emotional support helps individuals navigate the ups and downs of living with chronic pain and fosters a sense of connection and validation.
- Practical Assistance: Support networks can provide practical help with daily tasks and activities that may be challenging due to pain. This assistance can include help with household chores, transportation, and running errands,

which can alleviate the physical burden and stress of managing pain.

- Informational Resources: A support network can offer valuable information about managing chronic pain, including treatment options, coping strategies, and self-care techniques. Access to reliable information helps individuals make informed decisions about their care and explore various management approaches.
- Encouragement and Motivation: Support networks offer encouragement and motivation, which can be crucial for maintaining a positive outlook and staying engaged in self-care activities. Encouragement from others helps individuals remain resilient and committed to their pain management goals.

2. Building a Support Network
Concept and Steps:

Building a support network involves identifying and cultivating relationships with individuals and groups that can provide meaningful support. This process requires proactive efforts to establish and maintain connections, as well as to seek out resources that align with one's needs and preferences.

- Identifying Key Support Figures: Begin by identifying individuals in your life who can offer support, such as family members, friends, and colleagues. Consider people who are empathetic, understanding, and willing to provide assistance. Open communication with these individuals about your needs and how they can help is essential for building a strong support system.

- Engaging with Support Groups: Joining support groups, either in-person or online, can provide a valuable sense of community and connection with others who are experiencing similar challenges. Support groups offer opportunities to share experiences, exchange advice, and receive emotional support from people who truly understand the impact of chronic pain.

- Connecting with Healthcare Providers: Establishing a relationship with healthcare providers who are knowledgeable about chronic pain can enhance your support network. Healthcare professionals, including pain specialists, physical therapists, and mental health counselors, can provide expert guidance, treatment, and encouragement throughout your pain management journey.

- Utilizing Online Communities: Online communities and forums offer additional avenues for connecting with others who share similar experiences. These platforms allow individuals to seek advice, share stories, and find support from a diverse group of people who may be facing similar challenges.

- Building Relationships with Others in Pain: Connecting with others who have chronic pain can be particularly beneficial. They can provide insights, share coping strategies, and offer empathy based on their own experiences. Building relationships with peers who understand the daily realities of living with chronic pain can be deeply validating and supportive.

3. Maintaining and Nurturing Your Support Network

Concept and Strategies:

Maintaining and nurturing a support network requires ongoing effort and communication. Ensuring that your network remains strong and supportive involves regular engagement, expressing gratitude, and being open to giving and receiving support.

- Regular Communication: Keep in touch with your support network through regular communication, whether via phone calls, messages, or in-person visits. Sharing updates about your condition, expressing needs, and providing feedback helps maintain a strong and supportive relationship.
- Expressing Gratitude: Show appreciation for the support you receive from others. Expressing gratitude and acknowledging the efforts of those who help you reinforces positive relationships and encourages continued support.

- Being Supportive in Return: A strong support network is built on mutual support. Offer assistance and encouragement to others in your network when possible. Being there for others fosters reciprocal relationships and strengthens the sense of community and connection.

- Adjusting Support as Needed: As your needs and circumstances change, communicate any adjustments needed in your support network. Flexibility and open dialogue ensure that your network continues to meet your evolving needs and preferences.

- Seeking New Connections: Continuously seek opportunities to expand and enrich your support network. Engaging in new activities, joining additional groups, or reaching out to new individuals can provide fresh sources of support and perspective.

4. Leveraging Support Network for Specific Needs
Concept and Application:
Different aspects of managing chronic pain may require specific types of support. Leveraging your support network effectively involves identifying and utilizing the right resources for your particular needs.

- Crisis Situations: During periods of heightened pain or emotional distress, rely on your support network for immediate assistance. This may include seeking help with urgent tasks, emotional support, or professional guidance.
- Treatment Adherence: Utilize your network to stay motivated and adhere to treatment plans. Encouragement from family and friends can help you remain committed to your prescribed therapies and self-care routines.
- Educational Support: Engage with your network to gain insights and information about managing chronic pain. Leverage connections with healthcare professionals, support groups, and online communities to stay informed and make educated decisions.
- Social Engagement: Incorporate social activities into your routine to maintain connections and prevent isolation. Engage with your support network in enjoyable and meaningful activities that foster social interaction and positive experiences.

CHAPTER 8
MEDICATIONS AND ALTERNATIVE THERAPIES

OVERVIEW OF COMMON MEDICATIONS

Managing chronic pain often involves a combination of medications and alternative therapies to alleviate symptoms and improve quality of life. Understanding the various classes of medications used for pain management, their mechanisms of action, potential side effects, and appropriate usage is crucial for effective treatment. This section provides an extensive overview of common medications prescribed for chronic pain, categorized by their purpose and effects.

1. Analgesics
Definition and Purpose:
Analgesics are medications specifically designed to relieve pain. They work by modifying the pain signals sent to the brain or altering the perception of pain. Analgesics are typically categorized into two main types: non-opioid and opioid.

- **Non-Opioid Analgesics:** These include medications such as acetaminophen and nonsteroidal anti-inflammatory drugs (NSAIDs). Non-opioid analgesics are generally used for mild to moderate pain and are available over-the-counter or by prescription.

- **Acetaminophen (Tylenol):** Acetaminophen is a common over-the-counter pain reliever used for various types of pain, including headaches, muscle aches, and osteoarthritis. It works by inhibiting the production of prostaglandins in the brain, reducing pain and fever. While it is effective for pain relief, it does not have anti-inflammatory properties and can cause liver damage if used in excess.

- **NSAIDs (Ibuprofen, Naproxen, Aspirin):** NSAIDs work by reducing inflammation, which in turn alleviates pain. They are used for conditions such as arthritis, menstrual cramps, and back pain. By inhibiting cyclooxygenase (COX) enzymes, NSAIDs reduce the production of prostaglandins, which are chemicals involved in inflammation and pain. Long-term use of NSAIDs can lead to gastrointestinal issues, kidney damage, and increased risk of cardiovascular events.

- **Opioid Analgesics:** Opioids are potent pain relievers prescribed for moderate to severe pain that is not adequately controlled by non-opioid medications. They work by binding to opioid receptors in the brain and spinal cord, altering the perception of pain.

- **Examples**: Common opioids include morphine, oxycodone, hydrocodone, and fentanyl. These medications can be highly effective for short-term pain relief but carry a risk of dependence, addiction, and other side effects such as constipation, drowsiness, and nausea. Due to these risks, opioids are typically prescribed with caution and are usually considered a last resort after other pain management strategies have been explored.

2. Adjuvant Medications
Definition and Purpose:
Adjuvant medications are drugs that are not primarily designed to relieve pain but can be effective in managing chronic pain, especially when combined with other treatments. They are often used to enhance the effects of primary pain medications or to treat specific types of pain.

- **Antidepressants**: Certain antidepressants, particularly tricyclic antidepressants (TCAs) and serotonin-norepinephrine reuptake inhibitors (SNRIs), are used to treat chronic pain conditions such as fibromyalgia and neuropathic pain. These medications work by altering the levels of neurotransmitters in the brain, which can help modulate pain signals.
- **Examples**: Amitriptyline (a TCA) and Duloxetine (an SNRI) are commonly prescribed for pain management. They can help improve mood and sleep, which are often

disrupted by chronic pain. However, they may cause side effects like dry mouth, weight gain, and dizziness.

- **Anticonvulsants**: Anticonvulsants, primarily used to manage seizures, have also been found to be effective for neuropathic pain. They work by stabilizing nerve activity and preventing abnormal nerve firing that contributes to pain.

> - Examples: Gabapentin and Pregabalin are frequently used to treat nerve pain associated with conditions like diabetic neuropathy and postherpetic neuralgia. Potential side effects include dizziness, drowsiness, and swelling.

- Muscle Relaxants: These medications are used to relieve muscle spasms and associated pain. They work by relaxing the muscles and reducing muscle tension.

> - Examples: Baclofen, Cyclobenzaprine, and Tizanidine are common muscle relaxants prescribed for conditions involving muscle pain and spasms. Side effects can include drowsiness, dizziness, and muscle weakness.

3. Topical Medications
Definition and Purpose:
Topical medications are applied directly to the skin over the painful area. They are used for localized pain relief and can be effective for conditions such as arthritis and muscle strains.

- Topical Analgesics: These include creams, gels, and patches that contain active ingredients to relieve pain through the skin.

- Examples: Capsaicin cream, which contains a compound found in hot peppers, can reduce pain by depleting substance P, a neurotransmitter involved in pain signaling. Lidocaine patches contain a local anesthetic that temporarily numbs the area of application. Topical NSAIDs, such as diclofenac gel, can provide localized relief from pain and inflammation with fewer systemic side effects.

4. Combination Medications

Definition and Purpose:

Combination medications contain a mix of different types of drugs to enhance pain relief and reduce the need for higher doses of each component. These medications can provide a synergistic effect, improving pain management while potentially minimizing side effects.

- Examples: Combination products such as acetaminophen with codeine or hydrocodone with acetaminophen are designed to provide enhanced pain relief by combining an opioid with a non-opioid analgesic. These combinations can be effective for managing moderate to severe pain but require careful monitoring to avoid issues such as overdose and dependency.

5. Medication Management and Monitoring

Concept and Practice:

Effective pain management often involves careful monitoring and management of medications to ensure optimal efficacy and minimize risks. This includes regular assessment of medication effectiveness, adjustment of dosages, and monitoring for side effects.

- Regular Evaluation: Patients should have regular follow-ups with their healthcare providers to evaluate the effectiveness of their pain medications, assess any side effects, and make necessary adjustments. This ensures that the treatment remains effective and that potential issues are addressed promptly.

- Adjusting Dosages: Based on the patient's response to treatment and any changes in their condition, dosages may need to be adjusted. Healthcare providers may increase, decrease, or switch medications to find the most appropriate balance for managing pain while minimizing side effects.

- Monitoring for Side Effects: Patients should be aware of potential side effects associated with their medications and report any adverse reactions to their healthcare provider. This includes monitoring for symptoms such as gastrointestinal issues, mood changes, or signs of dependence and addiction.

ALTERNATIVE AND COMPLEMENTARY THERAPIES

Alternative and complementary therapies offer additional avenues for managing chronic pain, often used alongside conventional medical treatments. These therapies are based on various philosophies and practices, each aiming to improve pain management through different mechanisms. This section explores several widely recognized alternative and complementary therapies, their benefits, and how they can be integrated into a comprehensive pain management plan.

1. Acupuncture
Definition and Philosophy:
Acupuncture is a traditional Chinese medicine practice that involves inserting thin needles into specific points on the body to stimulate energy flow, known as Qi (pronounced "chee"). According to traditional Chinese medicine, disruptions in the flow of Qi can cause pain and other health issues. By targeting specific acupuncture points, practitioners aim to restore balance and improve the body's natural healing processes.
Mechanism of Action:

- Pain Relief: Acupuncture is believed to help reduce pain by stimulating the release of endorphins, the body's natural painkillers. It may also influence the nervous system to modulate pain signals and promote healing.
- Studies and Evidence: Research indicates that acupuncture can be effective for various types of chronic pain, including back pain, osteoarthritis, and migraines. While results can vary, many studies support its use as a complementary therapy for pain management.

Practitioner Qualifications and Safety:

- Certification: It is essential to seek treatment from a licensed and certified acupuncturist to ensure safety and efficacy. Practitioners should be trained in proper needle techniques and hygiene practices.
- Side Effects: Acupuncture is generally considered safe when performed by a trained professional. However, potential side effects can include minor bleeding, bruising, or temporary soreness at the needle sites.

2. Chiropractic Care

Definition and Philosophy:

Chiropractic care focuses on diagnosing and treating musculoskeletal disorders, particularly those related to the spine. Chiropractors use manual adjustments to align the spine and improve function, which is believed to enhance the body's ability to heal itself and relieve pain.

Mechanism of Action:

- Spinal Adjustments: Chiropractors perform spinal manipulations to correct misalignments, which may help alleviate pain by improving joint mobility and reducing nerve irritation.
- Evidence and Benefits: Research supports the effectiveness of chiropractic adjustments for certain conditions, such as acute lower back pain and tension headaches. However, its efficacy for other types of chronic pain remains debated.

Practitioner Qualifications and Safety:

- Certification: Chiropractors should be licensed and trained in spinal manipulation techniques. They may also use other modalities, such as exercise therapy or massage.
- Side Effects: Chiropractic care is generally safe, but some individuals may experience temporary soreness or discomfort following adjustments.

3. Massage Therapy

Definition and Philosophy:

Massage therapy involves manipulating the soft tissues of the body to improve circulation, reduce muscle tension, and promote relaxation. Different massage techniques, such as Swedish, deep tissue, and trigger point massage, are used based on the individual's needs and preferences.

Mechanism of Action:

- Muscle Relaxation: Massage therapy helps reduce muscle tension, which can alleviate pain and improve range of motion. It also stimulates the release of endorphins and promotes relaxation.
- Evidence and Benefits: Massage therapy has been shown to be effective for managing conditions such as chronic muscle pain, fibromyalgia, and stress-related pain. It can also enhance overall well-being and reduce anxiety.

Practitioner Qualifications and Safety:

- Certification: It is important to choose a licensed and trained massage therapist to ensure effective and safe treatment. Therapists should have training in various massage techniques and an understanding of anatomy.
- Side Effects: Most people experience only mild soreness after a massage. However, individuals with certain medical conditions or injuries should consult their healthcare provider before undergoing massage therapy.

4. Herbal and Nutritional Supplements

Definition and Philosophy:

Herbal and nutritional supplements are used to support health and manage chronic pain through natural means. They include a variety of products, such as herbs, vitamins, minerals, and other dietary supplements that may have anti-inflammatory, analgesic, or general health-promoting properties.

Common Supplements:

- Turmeric/Curcumin: Turmeric contains curcumin, which has anti-inflammatory properties and may help reduce pain associated with arthritis and other inflammatory conditions.
- Omega-3 Fatty Acids: Found in fish oil, omega-3 fatty acids have anti-inflammatory effects and may benefit individuals with chronic pain conditions like rheumatoid arthritis.
- Glucosamine and Chondroitin: These supplements are often used to support joint health and may help alleviate pain from osteoarthritis.

Evidence and Safety:

- Research and Effectiveness: Some supplements have shown promise in managing chronic pain, but results can vary. It is important to review scientific evidence and consult with a healthcare provider before using supplements.
- Interactions and Side Effects: Supplements can interact with medications and have potential side effects. Proper dosage and quality control are crucial to ensure safety and efficacy.

5. Mind-Body Practices

Definition and Philosophy:

Mind-body practices integrate mental and physical exercises to promote overall well-being and manage chronic pain. These practices emphasize the connection between the mind and body, aiming to enhance self-awareness, relaxation, and stress management.

Examples and Benefits:

- Yoga: Yoga combines physical postures, breathing exercises, and meditation to improve flexibility, strength, and relaxation. It has been shown to benefit individuals with chronic pain by reducing muscle tension and enhancing mental resilience.
- Tai Chi: Tai Chi is a form of gentle martial arts that involves slow, flowing movements and deep breathing. It can improve balance, reduce stress, and provide pain relief for conditions like arthritis.
- Biofeedback: Biofeedback uses electronic sensors to help individuals learn to control physiological functions, such as heart rate and muscle tension. It can be useful for managing stress and chronic pain by increasing awareness and self-regulation.

Practitioner Qualifications and Safety:

- Certification: Practitioners should be trained and certified in their respective mind-body practices. It is essential to work with professionals who have expertise in these techniques and can provide appropriate guidance.

- Side Effects: Mind-body practices are generally safe and have few side effects. However, individuals with specific health conditions should consult their healthcare provider before starting new practices.

6. Integrating Alternative Therapies

Concept and Practice:

Integrating alternative therapies into a chronic pain management plan involves combining them with conventional treatments to create a holistic approach. Collaboration between healthcare providers and practitioners of alternative therapies ensures that the chosen therapies complement existing treatments and address the individual's specific needs.

Considerations for Integration:

- Personalization: Tailor alternative therapies to individual preferences, health conditions, and pain management goals. What works for one person may not be effective for another.

- Communication with Healthcare Providers: Keep all healthcare providers informed about the use of alternative therapies to avoid potential interactions and ensure a coordinated approach to pain management.

- Monitoring and Evaluation: Regularly assess the effectiveness of alternative therapies and make adjustments as needed. This includes evaluating any improvements in pain levels, functional ability, and overall well-being.

EVALUATING TREATMENT OPTIONS

Evaluating treatment options is a critical component of managing chronic pain effectively. It involves assessing the benefits, risks, and suitability of various therapies to create a personalized pain management plan. This process requires a thorough understanding of each treatment option, its potential impact on the individual's condition, and how it aligns with their overall health goals.

1. Assessing Conventional Medications
Types of Medications:
- Analgesics: Analgesics, including over-the-counter options like acetaminophen and prescription opioids, are commonly used to manage pain. Their effectiveness varies depending on the type and severity of pain. It is essential to evaluate their effectiveness, potential side effects, and risk of dependency or abuse.
- Nonsteroidal Anti-Inflammatory Drugs (NSAIDs): NSAIDs, such as ibuprofen and naproxen, are used to reduce inflammation and pain. Assessing their long-term use involves understanding potential gastrointestinal, renal, and cardiovascular risks.

- Antidepressants and Anticonvulsants: These medications, often used for neuropathic pain, can have significant benefits but also potential side effects. Evaluating their impact involves monitoring mood changes, sleep patterns, and other symptoms.

Effectiveness and Side Effects:
- Efficacy: Evaluate how well each medication controls pain and improves quality of life. This includes assessing the degree of pain relief, functional improvements, and overall satisfaction with the treatment.
- Side Effects: Consider the potential side effects and how they affect daily living. For example, opioids may cause drowsiness or constipation, while NSAIDs can lead to stomach ulcers or kidney issues.

Monitoring and Adjustments:
- Regular Reviews: Regularly review the effectiveness and safety of medications. Adjust dosages or switch medications as needed to balance pain relief with minimizing side effects.
- Patient Feedback: Gather patient feedback on their experiences with medications, including any adverse effects or changes in pain levels. This information is crucial for making informed decisions about treatment adjustments.

2. Evaluating Alternative and Complementary Therapies

Types of Therapies:

- Acupuncture and Chiropractic Care: Assess the effectiveness of these therapies in managing pain and improving overall function. Consider factors such as the frequency of treatments, costs, and any immediate or long-term benefits.
- Massage Therapy and Herbal Supplements: Evaluate the benefits and any potential interactions with other treatments. Review scientific evidence supporting their use and discuss any reported improvements or side effects.

Evidence and Research:

- Scientific Studies: Examine the evidence from clinical studies and research to determine the efficacy of alternative therapies. This includes looking at randomized controlled trials, meta-analyses, and patient testimonials.
- Quality and Safety: Ensure that alternative therapies are performed by qualified practitioners and that supplements meet quality standards. Safety is a key consideration, especially when combining alternative therapies with conventional treatments.

Integration into Pain Management Plan:

- Combination Therapies: Evaluate how alternative therapies can be integrated with conventional treatments to enhance overall pain management. This may involve combining therapies to address different aspects of pain or using them as complementary approaches.

- Personalization: Tailor alternative therapies to individual needs, preferences, and health conditions. What works for one person may not be effective for another, so personalized treatment plans are essential.

3. Considering Lifestyle and Self-Care Approaches

Lifestyle Modifications:

- Exercise and Physical Activity: Assess the role of exercise in managing pain and improving function. Consider factors such as the type, frequency, and intensity of physical activity, and its impact on pain levels and overall health.

- Diet and Nutrition: Evaluate the influence of dietary changes on pain management. Consider the benefits of anti-inflammatory foods and any dietary adjustments that may improve overall well-being.

Self-Care Strategies:

- Mindfulness and Stress Management: Assess the effectiveness of mindfulness techniques, such as meditation and relaxation exercises, in managing pain and stress. Review their impact on overall quality of life and emotional well-being.

- Self-Monitoring and Adjustment: Encourage individuals to track their pain levels, treatment responses, and any changes in symptoms. This information is valuable for adjusting treatment plans and making informed decisions.

Support Systems:

- Building a Support Network: Evaluate the importance of social support and how it contributes to pain management. Consider the role of family, friends, and support groups in providing emotional and practical support.
- Professional Support: Assess the need for professional support, such as counseling or therapy, to address the psychological aspects of chronic pain. Review the benefits of working with mental health professionals to manage stress, anxiety, and depression.

4. Making Informed Decisions

Informed Choice:

- Patient Education: Ensure that patients are well-informed about their treatment options, including potential benefits, risks, and side effects. Provide clear and accurate information to help patients make informed decisions about their care.
- Shared Decision-Making: Involve patients in the decision-making process by discussing their preferences, goals, and concerns. Collaborative

decision-making ensures that treatment plans align with patients' values and priorities.

Ongoing Evaluation:

- Regular Follow-Up: Schedule regular follow-up appointments to assess the effectiveness of treatment options and make necessary adjustments. Monitor changes in pain levels, functional abilities, and overall quality of life.

- Feedback and Adaptation: Continuously gather feedback from patients and adapt treatment plans based on their experiences and evolving needs. This approach ensures that treatment remains effective and responsive to changes in their condition.

DISCUSSING TREATMENTS WITH YOUR HEALTHCARE PROVIDER

Engaging in a thorough and open dialogue with your healthcare provider about treatment options is essential for effective pain management. This discussion ensures that you are well-informed, involved in decision-making, and able to address any concerns or preferences you may have regarding your treatment plan. This section provides guidance on how to approach these conversations, what information to consider, and how to maximize the benefits of your interactions with healthcare professionals.

1. Preparing for the Discussion
Gather Relevant Information:
- Medical History: Prepare a comprehensive summary of your medical history, including previous treatments, current medications, allergies, and any other health conditions. This information helps your provider understand your overall health context and tailor recommendations accordingly.
- Pain History and Symptoms: Document your pain history, including the onset, duration, intensity, and any factors that exacerbate or alleviate your pain. Include details on how pain impacts your daily life, functional abilities, and emotional well-being.
- Treatment Goals and Preferences: Reflect on your goals for treatment, such as pain reduction, improved function, or enhanced quality of life. Consider your preferences for different types of treatments, including conventional medications, alternative therapies, or lifestyle modifications.

List Questions and Concerns:
- Questions About Options: Prepare a list of questions about the different treatment options available. This may include inquiries about

effectiveness, potential side effects, duration of treatment, and any required lifestyle changes.

- Concerns About Risks and Benefits: Identify any concerns you have about the risks or benefits of specific treatments. Discuss how these risks align with your overall health goals and what measures can be taken to mitigate potential adverse effects.

2. Engaging in the Conversation

Communicate Openly and Honestly:

- Describe Your Experience: Share detailed information about your pain experiences, including how they affect your daily activities and quality of life. Be honest about any challenges or limitations you encounter with current treatments.
- Express Your Preferences: Clearly communicate your preferences for treatment options, including any alternative or complementary therapies you are interested in exploring. Discuss any reservations you may have about conventional treatments and why.

Discuss Treatment Options:

- Review Each Option: Go over each treatment option with your provider, discussing the potential benefits, risks, and how each option aligns with your goals. Ask for explanations of how specific treatments work and their expected outcomes.

- Evaluate Evidence: Request information on the scientific evidence supporting each treatment option. Discuss clinical studies, research findings, and any relevant patient testimonials that may inform your decision.

Consider the Integration of Therapies:

- Combination Approaches: Explore the possibility of combining different therapies to address various aspects of your pain management. For example, you might discuss integrating physical therapy with pharmacological treatments or incorporating mindfulness techniques alongside medication.
- Personalized Plans: Work with your provider to create a personalized treatment plan that takes into account your specific needs, preferences, and health goals. Ensure that the plan is adaptable and can be modified based on your responses to treatments.

3. Addressing Concerns and Making Decisions

Discuss Potential Side Effects:

- Understanding Risks: Have a thorough discussion about the potential side effects of each treatment option. Consider how these side effects might impact your daily life and any steps that can be taken to manage or minimize them.
- Risk Management: Explore strategies for managing risks associated with treatments, such

as monitoring for adverse effects, adjusting dosages, or seeking additional support from healthcare professionals.

Evaluate Treatment Duration and Adjustments:

- Treatment Timeline: Discuss the expected duration of each treatment option and what milestones or markers will be used to assess its effectiveness. Understand how long it will take to see results and what to expect during this period.
- Adjustments and Flexibility: Consider how the treatment plan can be adjusted based on your progress and changing needs. Discuss how frequently you will need follow-up appointments to review and modify the plan as necessary.

Involve Family and Support System:

- Family Discussions: If relevant, involve family members or caregivers in the discussion about treatment options. Their support and understanding can be valuable in implementing and adhering to the treatment plan.
- Support System: Utilize your support system to help you make informed decisions and to provide encouragement throughout the treatment process.

4. Following Up and Monitoring

Regular Follow-Up Appointments:

- Schedule Reviews: Set up regular follow-up appointments to monitor your progress and discuss any changes in your condition or response to treatments. These appointments are crucial for assessing the effectiveness of the treatment plan and making necessary adjustments.

- Track Progress: Keep track of your pain levels, functional abilities, and any changes in symptoms between appointments. Share this information with your provider to help guide decision-making and treatment adjustments.

Feedback and Communication:

- Provide Feedback: Offer feedback on your experiences with the treatment plan, including any improvements or challenges. Your input helps your provider understand how well the plan is working and what modifications may be needed.
- Ongoing Communication: Maintain open lines of communication with your healthcare provider throughout your treatment journey. Address any new concerns, questions, or issues as they arise to ensure a collaborative approach to pain management.

Adapting to Changes:

- Responsive Adjustments: Be prepared to adapt your treatment plan based on changes in your condition, new research findings, or evolving needs. Work with your provider to make informed adjustments that continue to align with your goals and preferences.

CHAPTER 9
MONITORING PROGRESS AND ADJUSTING YOUR PLAN

TRACKING PAIN AND PROGRESS

Effective management of chronic pain requires a systematic approach to monitoring and evaluating both pain levels and overall progress. This involves using various tools and methods to collect data on pain intensity, functional limitations, and treatment efficacy. Tracking progress allows individuals and healthcare providers to make informed decisions about treatment adjustments, ensuring that the pain management plan remains effective and responsive to changing needs.

1. Methods for Tracking Pain
Pain Diaries and Journals:

- Daily Entries: Maintain a daily pain diary or journal to record details about pain intensity, duration, and location. Note any factors that may influence pain levels, such as activities, stress, or dietary changes. This detailed record helps identify patterns and triggers that can inform treatment adjustments.

- Severity Scales: Use standardized pain severity scales, such as the Numeric Rating Scale (NRS) or the Visual Analog Scale (VAS), to quantify pain levels. Regularly documenting pain scores provides objective data that can be useful for assessing treatment effectiveness.

Electronic Tracking Tools:

- Pain Management Apps: Utilize mobile apps designed for tracking pain and symptoms. These apps often include features for logging pain levels, medication use, and other relevant factors. They can generate visual charts and reports to help identify trends over time.
- Wearable Devices: Explore wearable devices that monitor physiological indicators related to pain, such as activity levels, sleep patterns, and heart rate. These devices can provide valuable insights into how pain affects daily activities and overall well-being.

Regular Assessments:

- Scheduled Evaluations: Schedule regular assessments with your healthcare provider to review pain levels and progress. These evaluations may include physical examinations, questionnaires, and discussions about any changes in symptoms or treatment responses.
- Self-Assessment Tools: Use validated self-assessment tools, such as the Brief Pain

Inventory (BPI) or the McGill Pain Questionnaire, to evaluate pain characteristics and impact. These tools can provide a comprehensive overview of how pain affects various aspects of life.

2. Monitoring Functional Abilities

Daily Functionality Assessments:

- Activity Logs: Keep a log of daily activities and their impact on pain levels. Document how specific activities, such as work tasks, household chores, or recreational activities, affect pain intensity and functional abilities.
- Functional Limitations: Track any limitations in physical function, such as difficulty with mobility, strength, or endurance. Note changes in your ability to perform daily tasks and engage in social or recreational activities.

Quality of Life Measures:

- Overall Well-Being: Assess the impact of pain on overall quality of life, including physical, emotional, and social aspects. Use quality of life questionnaires, such as the SF-36 or the PROMIS (Patient-Reported Outcomes Measurement Information System), to evaluate how pain affects your well-being.
- Emotional Impact: Monitor any changes in mood, stress levels, and emotional well-being. Chronic pain can significantly affect mental

health, so tracking these aspects is important for a holistic approach to pain management.

Functional Goals:

- Goal Setting: Establish specific, measurable, achievable, relevant, and time-bound (SMART) goals for improving functional abilities. Regularly review progress toward these goals and adjust them as needed based on changes in pain levels and functional status.
- Progress Reviews: Evaluate progress toward functional goals during follow-up appointments with your healthcare provider. Discuss any barriers or challenges encountered and develop strategies to overcome them.

3. Adjusting the Treatment Plan

Evaluating Treatment Effectiveness:

- Effectiveness Review: Assess the effectiveness of current treatments based on pain tracking data and functional assessments. Determine whether the treatments are achieving the desired outcomes, such as pain relief, improved function, or enhanced quality of life.
- Side Effects Monitoring: Review any side effects or adverse reactions experienced with current treatments. Consider how these side effects impact overall well-being and whether they warrant adjustments to the treatment plan.

Making Adjustments:

- Treatment Modifications: Based on progress and feedback, make adjustments to the treatment plan as needed. This may involve altering medication dosages, changing therapies, or incorporating new interventions.
- Combining Therapies: Explore the possibility of combining different treatment approaches to address various aspects of pain management. For example, you might integrate physical therapy with pharmacological treatments or combine mindfulness techniques with medication.

Collaborative Decision-Making:

- Engaging with Your Provider: Work closely with your healthcare provider to review progress, discuss treatment options, and make informed decisions about adjustments. Share your experiences, preferences, and any concerns to ensure a collaborative approach.
- Patient Involvement: Actively participate in the decision-making process by providing feedback on treatment responses and discussing any changes in symptoms or functional abilities. Your involvement is crucial for developing a personalized and effective pain management plan.

4. Long-Term Monitoring and Adaptation

Continuous Monitoring:

- Ongoing Tracking: Continue tracking pain levels, functional abilities, and treatment responses over the long term. Regular monitoring helps identify any new patterns or changes in pain management needs.

- Adapting to Changes: Be prepared to adapt the treatment plan in response to evolving needs, such as changes in pain intensity, new symptoms, or shifts in functional status. Regular follow-ups with your healthcare provider are essential for making timely adjustments.

Reviewing and Updating Goals:

- Goal Reevaluation: Periodically review and update functional goals based on progress and any changes in your condition. Ensure that goals remain relevant and achievable as your pain management plan evolves.

- Long-Term Planning: Develop a long-term plan for managing chronic pain, incorporating strategies for ongoing monitoring, adjustment, and self-care. This plan should address both immediate and future needs, ensuring continued effectiveness and support.

ASSESSING THE EFFECTIVENESS OF YOUR PLAN

Evaluating the effectiveness of a chronic pain management plan is crucial for ensuring that treatment strategies are achieving their intended goals and providing the desired relief. Regular assessment helps identify whether the current plan is successful, whether adjustments are needed, and how to optimize pain management for the best possible outcomes. This process involves a systematic review of treatment efficacy, side effects, functional improvements, and overall quality of life.

1. Evaluating Pain Relief
Quantifying Pain Reduction:
- Pain Scales and Diaries: Use pain scales, such as the Numeric Rating Scale (NRS) or Visual Analog Scale (VAS), to measure pain intensity regularly. Compare these measurements with baseline levels to assess the degree of pain reduction achieved with the current plan.
- Daily Pain Records: Maintain detailed records of daily pain experiences, noting any changes in pain intensity, frequency, and duration. Analyze these records to determine trends and evaluate the effectiveness of pain relief strategies.

Assessing Changes in Pain Patterns:

- Pain Fluctuations: Observe any fluctuations in pain patterns, such as periods of relief or worsening symptoms. Assess how these changes correlate with specific aspects of the treatment plan, such as medication adjustments or lifestyle modifications.
- Trigger Identification: Identify any new triggers or factors influencing pain levels, and evaluate whether the current plan effectively addresses these factors. Consider whether additional interventions are needed to manage newly identified triggers.

2. Monitoring Functional Improvements

Evaluating Functional Abilities:

- Daily Activities: Assess changes in your ability to perform daily activities and tasks. Consider how pain management strategies have impacted your functional capabilities, such as mobility, strength, and endurance.
- Functional Assessments: Use standardized functional assessments, such as the Oswestry Disability Index (ODI) or the Roland-Morris Disability Questionnaire, to evaluate improvements in physical function. Compare results over time to gauge the effectiveness of the treatment plan.

Setting and Reviewing Goals:

- Goal Achievement: Review progress toward specific functional goals established as part of the treatment plan. Determine whether these goals have been met and if they require adjustment based on your current status.
- Revised Goals: Based on functional improvements, update and set new goals as needed. Ensure that these goals remain realistic and aligned with your evolving needs and capabilities.

3. Assessing Side Effects and Tolerability

Identifying Adverse Effects:

- Side Effect Tracking: Monitor any side effects or adverse reactions associated with treatments, such as medications or therapies. Record the frequency, severity, and impact of these side effects on your daily life.
- Impact on Quality of Life: Evaluate how side effects affect your overall quality of life. Consider whether these effects outweigh the benefits of the treatment or if they necessitate adjustments to the treatment plan.

Evaluating Tolerability:

- Treatment Tolerability: Assess how well you tolerate various treatments, including their impact on your overall well-being and daily functioning.

Determine if there are any aspects of the plan that are particularly challenging or uncomfortable.

- Adjustments for Tolerability: Work with your healthcare provider to adjust treatments or explore alternative options if side effects become intolerable or negatively impact your quality of life.

4. Reviewing Overall Quality of Life

Quality of Life Measures:

- Self-Reported Assessments: Use quality of life questionnaires, such as the SF-36 or PROMIS, to evaluate the impact of chronic pain and treatment on your physical, emotional, and social well-being. These assessments provide a comprehensive view of how pain management affects your overall life.
- Holistic Evaluation: Consider other aspects of your life, such as sleep quality, mood, social interactions, and ability to engage in meaningful activities. Assess how well the treatment plan supports improvements in these areas.

Long-Term Impact:

- Sustained Improvement: Evaluate the long-term impact of the treatment plan on your quality of life. Assess whether improvements in pain relief and functional abilities are sustained over time and if they contribute to a better overall quality of life.

- Future Planning: Consider how the current plan aligns with your long-term goals and needs. Plan for future adjustments or additional interventions based on ongoing assessments and evolving life circumstances.

5. Gathering Feedback from Healthcare Providers

Healthcare Provider Reviews:

- Professional Assessments: Seek feedback from healthcare providers on the effectiveness of the treatment plan. Discuss any observations or recommendations they have based on their professional assessments and experience.
- Collaborative Review: Engage in collaborative reviews with your provider to evaluate treatment effectiveness, address any concerns, and make informed decisions about potential adjustments or alternative strategies.

Patient-Provider Communication:

- Regular Updates: Provide regular updates to your healthcare provider about your progress, including pain levels, functional improvements, and any new symptoms or issues. Ensure that your provider is fully informed to support effective decision-making.
- Discuss Adjustments: Use feedback from your provider to discuss potential adjustments to the treatment plan. Explore options for optimizing

pain management and addressing any challenges or concerns that arise.

6. Making Informed Adjustments

Analyzing Data:

- Review Collected Data: Analyze the data collected from pain diaries, functional assessments, and quality of life measures. Identify trends, patterns, and areas where the current plan is successful or lacking.
- Evidence-Based Decisions: Use evidence-based practices and clinical guidelines to inform decisions about treatment adjustments. Consider the latest research and best practices to guide modifications to the plan.

Implementing Changes:

- Adjust Treatment Strategies: Based on the assessment, implement necessary changes to the treatment plan. This may include modifying medication dosages, incorporating new therapies, or altering lifestyle interventions.
- Monitoring Results: After making adjustments, continue monitoring pain levels, functional abilities, and overall quality of life. Evaluate the impact of changes and refine the plan as needed to achieve optimal outcomes.

WHEN TO SEEK ADDITIONAL HELP

Knowing when to seek additional help is a critical aspect of managing chronic pain effectively. While self-management strategies and initial treatments often form the foundation of pain management, there are instances when professional intervention becomes necessary to address unresolved issues, adapt to changes, or explore advanced options. Recognizing the signs that indicate the need for further assistance can ensure timely and appropriate care, improving overall outcomes and quality of life.

1. Persistent or Worsening Pain
Ongoing Pain Despite Treatment:
- Unresponsive Pain: If you continue to experience significant pain despite adhering to your current treatment plan, it may indicate that the plan is not adequately addressing the underlying issues. Persistent pain may signal the need for a reassessment of your diagnosis or treatment approach.

- Increasing Pain Intensity: An increase in the intensity or frequency of pain can suggest that your condition is progressing or that the current management strategies are not effective. This change requires evaluation to adjust the treatment plan and explore alternative options.

New or Unusual Symptoms:

- Emergence of New Symptoms: The appearance of new or unusual symptoms, such as unexpected pain patterns, neurological changes, or other health issues, may warrant further investigation. These symptoms could be related to the underlying condition or side effects of treatment.
- Unexplained Symptoms: Symptoms that do not align with your known condition or that are difficult to explain should be evaluated by a healthcare professional to rule out complications or new health concerns.

2. Limited Improvement in Functionality

Impact on Daily Activities:

- Functional Limitations: If chronic pain continues to limit your ability to perform daily activities, work, or engage in social and recreational pursuits despite treatment efforts, it may be necessary to seek additional support. Improved functionality is a key goal of pain management, and limited progress may indicate a need for more comprehensive intervention.

- Difficulty Achieving Goals: When you struggle to meet the functional goals set as part of your treatment plan, despite making efforts and following recommendations, it may be time to consult with specialists to explore more effective strategies or therapies.

Changes in Physical Abilities:

- Decline in Physical Function: A noticeable decline in physical abilities, such as mobility, strength, or coordination, may require further evaluation. Changes in physical function can impact overall quality of life and may need targeted interventions to address underlying issues or optimize management strategies.

3. Side Effects or Adverse Reactions

Severe or Unmanageable Side Effects:

- Intolerable Side Effects: If you experience severe or intolerable side effects from medications or treatments, such as nausea, dizziness, or cognitive impairment, it is essential to seek additional help. Severe side effects can impact your daily life and may necessitate adjustments to your treatment plan or alternative therapies.

- Impact on Quality of Life: Side effects that significantly affect your quality of life, including mental health or social interactions, should be discussed with your healthcare provider.

Addressing these issues can help improve your overall well-being and treatment experience.

Allergic Reactions or Complications:

- Allergic Reactions: Allergic reactions to medications or therapies, such as rash, swelling, or breathing difficulties, require immediate medical attention. Prompt action is necessary to manage these reactions and avoid potentially serious complications.
- Complications from Treatments: Complications arising from treatments, such as infections from injections or injuries from physical therapies, need to be addressed to prevent further health issues and ensure effective pain management.

4. Psychological and Emotional Struggles

Mental Health Concerns:

- Emotional Distress: Persistent feelings of depression, anxiety, or emotional distress related to chronic pain may indicate a need for additional psychological support. Chronic pain often impacts mental health, and addressing these aspects is crucial for comprehensive management.
- Psychological Symptoms: If psychological symptoms, such as changes in mood, sleep disturbances, or cognitive issues, become severe or unmanageable, seeking help from mental

health professionals can provide valuable support and interventions.

Difficulty Coping with Pain:

- Coping Challenges: If you find it increasingly difficult to cope with the emotional and psychological aspects of chronic pain, additional help may be necessary. Support from therapists, counselors, or support groups can offer strategies and resources to improve coping mechanisms and emotional resilience.

5. Need for Specialized Care

Consultation with Specialists:

- Referral to Specialists: If your condition requires expertise beyond the scope of your primary healthcare provider, such as pain specialists, neurologists, or rheumatologists, seeking a referral to a specialist can provide targeted and advanced care options.
- Advanced Diagnostic Testing: Specialized diagnostic tests or imaging may be needed to further investigate complex pain conditions. Consulting with specialists can ensure that you receive comprehensive evaluations and appropriate treatment recommendations.

Exploring Advanced Treatments:

- Consideration of Advanced Therapies: If standard treatments have proven ineffective, exploring advanced or experimental therapies, such as nerve blocks, spinal cord stimulators, or multidisciplinary approaches, may be necessary. Specialists can guide you in accessing these treatments and assessing their suitability for your condition.

6. Impact on Overall Well-being

Quality of Life Evaluation:

- Overall Well-being: When chronic pain significantly impacts your overall quality of life, including social, occupational, and recreational aspects, additional help may be needed to address these broader issues. A multidisciplinary approach can provide holistic support and improve various aspects of well-being.
- Long-Term Management: For ongoing or worsening issues, working with healthcare providers to develop a long-term management plan that addresses all aspects of your health and well-being can be beneficial.

Life Changes and Adjustments:

- Major Life Changes: If significant life changes, such as changes in work status, personal relationships, or daily routines, impact your pain management, seeking guidance from healthcare providers or support services can help you adapt and maintain effective management strategies.

MAKING ADJUSTMENTS TO IMPROVE OUTCOMES

Making adjustments to your chronic pain management plan is essential for optimizing outcomes and ensuring that the strategies you employ remain effective over time. Chronic pain management is a dynamic process that requires regular review and modification based on ongoing experiences, changes in health status, and evolving needs. This section provides an in-depth exploration of how to make thoughtful and informed adjustments to improve your overall pain management outcomes.

1. Reviewing and Analyzing Current Strategies

Assessing Treatment Effectiveness:

- Evaluate Current Treatments: Regularly review the effectiveness of current treatments, including medications, therapies, and lifestyle changes. Assess whether these treatments are meeting your goals for pain relief, functionality, and quality of life.
- Monitor Side Effects: Keep track of any side effects or adverse reactions associated with your treatments. If side effects are significant or unmanageable, consider discussing alternatives or adjustments with your healthcare provider.

Analyzing Pain Patterns:

- Identify Pain Trends: Observe and document any patterns or changes in your pain levels. Understanding these trends can help identify triggers, fluctuations, or new symptoms that may require adjustments to your management plan.

- Review Impact on Daily Life: Assess how your pain affects your daily activities, work, and social interactions. Consider whether your current strategies are effectively addressing these impacts and making necessary adjustments to improve overall functioning.

2. Setting New Goals and Objectives

Revising Treatment Goals:

- Update Goals Based on Progress: Based on your ongoing assessments, update your treatment goals to reflect changes in your condition or improvements in your overall well-being. Set realistic and achievable objectives that align with your current needs and priorities.

- Adjust Functional Goals: Re-evaluate your functional goals, such as improvements in mobility, strength, or daily activity levels. Adjust these goals as needed to ensure that they are challenging yet attainable, and aligned with your overall treatment plan.

Incorporating New Objectives:

- Introduce New Goals: As you progress, consider introducing new objectives to address areas of your life that may still be impacted by pain. These could include improving specific physical abilities, enhancing mental well-being, or exploring new coping strategies.
- Focus on Long-Term Outcomes: Develop long-term objectives that reflect your desired outcomes for managing chronic pain. These goals should encompass not only pain relief but also improvements in overall quality of life, emotional well-being, and daily functioning.

3. Exploring New Treatment Options

Investigating Alternative Therapies:

- Explore New Therapies: If current treatments are not yielding the desired results, consider exploring alternative therapies or complementary approaches. These may include newer medications, innovative physical therapies, or emerging pain management techniques.
- Research Evidence-Based Options: Look for evidence-based treatments that have demonstrated effectiveness in managing chronic pain. Consult with healthcare professionals to determine whether these options are appropriate for your specific condition and needs.

Consulting with Specialists:

- Seek Specialist Opinions: If necessary, consult with specialists who can provide additional insights and recommendations for managing chronic pain. Specialists such as pain management experts, neurologists, or rheumatologists may offer new perspectives and treatment options.
- Consider Multidisciplinary Approaches: Explore multidisciplinary approaches that integrate various types of care, such as physical therapy, psychological support, and medical treatments. A comprehensive approach can enhance overall management and address multiple aspects of chronic pain.

4. Adjusting Self-Care and Lifestyle Modifications

Enhancing Self-Care Practices:

- Revise Self-Care Routines: Reassess your self-care practices, including diet, exercise, and stress management techniques. Make adjustments to enhance their effectiveness and ensure they align with your current needs and goals.
- Implement New Strategies: Incorporate new self-care strategies or modify existing ones to address areas where you may be struggling. This could involve adjusting your exercise routine, trying new relaxation techniques, or improving your nutritional habits.

Updating Lifestyle Modifications:

- Adapt Lifestyle Changes: Review any lifestyle changes you have implemented and evaluate their impact on your chronic pain. Adjust these changes as needed to better support your overall management plan and improve your quality of life.
- Balance Daily Activities: Ensure that your daily activities are balanced to avoid overexertion or underactivity. Adjust your schedule and routines to accommodate your pain levels and maintain a healthy balance between activity and rest.

5. Engaging in Regular Communication

Maintaining Open Dialogue:

- Communicate with Healthcare Providers: Maintain regular communication with your healthcare providers to discuss your progress, challenges, and any adjustments needed. Share updates on your pain levels, treatment effectiveness, and any new symptoms or concerns.
- Seek Feedback: Request feedback from your healthcare team on your progress and any modifications to your plan. Their insights and recommendations can guide you in making informed decisions and improving your overall management strategies.

Utilizing Support Networks:

- Involve Support Systems: Engage your support network, including family, friends, and caregivers, in your pain management plan. Their involvement can provide additional support, encouragement, and practical assistance as you make adjustments.

- Participate in Support Groups: Consider participating in support groups or forums where you can share experiences, gain insights, and receive support from others with similar conditions. These interactions can offer valuable perspectives and ideas for improving your management plan.

6. Monitoring and Documenting Adjustments

Tracking Changes:

- Document Adjustments: Keep detailed records of any changes made to your pain management plan, including new treatments, modifications to self-care practices, and updates to goals. Documentation helps track progress and assess the impact of adjustments.

- Evaluate Outcomes: Regularly review the outcomes of any changes made to your plan. Assess whether these adjustments have led to improvements in pain management, functionality, and overall well-being.

Reviewing Progress:

- Schedule Follow-Ups: Schedule regular follow-up appointments with your healthcare providers to review progress and discuss the effectiveness of recent adjustments. Use these opportunities to make further refinements to your plan as needed.
- Adapt Based on Results: Be prepared to make additional adjustments based on the results of your evaluations. Continuous adaptation ensures that your pain management plan remains responsive to your evolving needs and circumstances.

CHAPTER 10

FUTURE TRENDS AND RESEARCH

EMERGING TREATMENTS AND TECHNOLOGIES

The field of chronic pain management is continually evolving, with ongoing research and technological advancements paving the way for innovative treatments and therapies. This chapter explores the latest developments in emerging treatments and technologies, offering insights into how these advancements may shape the future of chronic pain management. Understanding these trends can provide patients, heal?thcare professionals, and researchers with valuable information about potential future directions and improvements in care.

1. Advancements in Pharmacological Treatments
Novel Drug Developments:

- New Drug Classes: Research is focused on developing new classes of medications that target different pain pathways or mechanisms. These include drugs designed to selectively modulate pain receptors or alter neurotransmitter levels in more precise ways, potentially offering more effective and targeted relief.

- Personalized Medicine: Advances in genomics and pharmacogenomics are driving the development of personalized pain medications. By analyzing genetic markers, researchers aim to tailor treatments to individual genetic profiles, enhancing efficacy and minimizing adverse effects.

Opioid Alternatives:

- Non-Opioid Analgesics: Efforts are underway to develop alternative analgesics that provide effective pain relief without the risks associated with opioid use. This includes research into non-opioid pain medications, such as novel anti-inflammatory drugs and compounds that modulate pain pathways differently.

- Biologics and Monoclonal Antibodies: Emerging biologic therapies, including monoclonal antibodies, are being investigated for their potential to target specific inflammatory processes or pain pathways with high precision. These treatments aim to reduce pain while minimizing systemic side effects.

2. Innovations in Physical Therapy and Rehabilitation

Advanced Physical Therapy Techniques:

- Technology-Enhanced Therapy: The integration of technology into physical therapy is offering new ways to improve rehabilitation outcomes. Virtual reality (VR) and augmented reality (AR) systems are being used to create immersive therapy environments that enhance patient engagement and provide real-time feedback on movements.

- Robotics and Exoskeletons: Robotic-assisted therapy and wearable exoskeletons are being developed to support patients with chronic pain in improving mobility and strength. These technologies offer precise, controlled movements and can be tailored to individual needs for effective rehabilitation.

Telehealth and Remote Monitoring:

- Telephysical Therapy: Remote physical therapy sessions are becoming more common, allowing patients to receive guided exercise routines and therapy from their homes. Telehealth platforms enable therapists to monitor progress and provide feedback in real time.
- Wearable Sensors: Wearable technology, including smart sensors and fitness trackers, is being used to monitor physical activity and movement patterns. These devices can provide valuable data for customizing rehabilitation programs and tracking progress.

3. Advances in Mind-Body Interventions

Mindfulness-Based Therapies:

- Neuroscientific Research: Research into the neurobiological effects of mindfulness and meditation is expanding, offering insights into how these practices can alter brain function and pain perception. Studies are exploring how mindfulness-based therapies can enhance pain management and improve emotional resilience.

- Innovative Programs: New mindfulness and cognitive-behavioral programs are being developed to address chronic pain through digital platforms. Apps and online programs provide accessible tools for practicing mindfulness and stress reduction.

Integrative Approaches:

- Holistic Therapies: The integration of holistic approaches, such as acupuncture, massage therapy, and biofeedback, is gaining attention for their potential benefits in managing chronic pain. Research is focused on understanding how these therapies can be combined with conventional treatments to enhance overall care.

- Personalized Mind-Body Approaches: Tailored mind-body interventions that consider individual preferences and needs are being explored. These approaches aim to personalize therapy based on patient characteristics, pain types, and psychological factors.

4. Cutting-Edge Research in Pain Mechanisms

Genetic and Molecular Research:

- Genetic Studies: Advances in genetic research are uncovering the genetic underpinnings of chronic pain conditions. Studies are identifying genetic variants associated with pain sensitivity, progression, and response to treatment, which may lead to more targeted therapies.
- Molecular Mechanisms: Research into the molecular mechanisms of pain is revealing new targets for treatment. Understanding the role of specific molecules, such as cytokines and neurotransmitters, in pain pathways can lead to the development of novel therapeutic agents.

Neuroplasticity and Pain Modulation:

- Neuroplasticity Research: Investigations into neuroplasticity—the brain's ability to reorganize itself in response to pain—are providing insights into how chronic pain alters brain function. This research may lead to interventions that can modify pain-related neural circuits and improve pain management.
- Pain Modulation Techniques: Emerging techniques for modulating pain perception, such as transcranial magnetic stimulation (TMS) and deep brain stimulation (DBS), are being studied for their potential to provide relief for chronic pain conditions by targeting specific brain regions involved in pain processing.

5. Future Directions in Chronic Pain Management

Integrated Care Models:

- Multidisciplinary Approaches: The future of chronic pain management is likely to involve more integrated care models that combine various disciplines, including pain specialists, physical therapists, psychologists, and complementary medicine practitioners. These models aim to address the multifaceted nature of chronic pain and provide comprehensive care.
- Patient-Centered Care: A growing emphasis on patient-centered care is expected to shape future treatment approaches. This includes involving patients in decision-making, tailoring treatments to individual needs, and prioritizing patient preferences and goals in the management plan.

Innovative Technology Applications:

- Artificial Intelligence: The use of artificial intelligence (AI) and machine learning in pain management is being explored to analyze large datasets, predict treatment outcomes, and personalize care. AI may enhance diagnostic accuracy and support the development of customized treatment plans.
- Digital Health Solutions: The expansion of digital health solutions, such as mobile health apps and online platforms, is likely to continue. These tools provide patients with resources for

self-management, tracking progress, and accessing support.

CURRENT RESEARCH IN CHRONIC PAIN MANAGEMENT

Current research in chronic pain management is focused on advancing our understanding of pain mechanisms, improving treatment options, and developing innovative approaches to enhance patient care. This section delves into the latest research findings, highlighting key areas of exploration and their potential impact on chronic pain management. By examining these research endeavors, we gain insights into the evolving landscape of pain management and future possibilities for effective interventions.

1. Understanding Pain Mechanisms

Neurobiological Research:

- Pain Pathways: Researchers are continually investigating the neural pathways involved in chronic pain, including the central and peripheral nervous systems. This includes studying the role of specific brain regions, spinal cord pathways, and neurotransmitter systems in pain perception and modulation. Understanding these pathways can reveal new targets for therapeutic intervention and inform the development of more effective treatments.

- Neuroinflammation: Recent studies have focused on the role of neuroinflammation in chronic pain. Neuroinflammation refers to the inflammatory response within the nervous system, which can contribute to pain sensitivity and persistence. Research is exploring how inflammatory processes in the brain and spinal cord influence pain and how targeting these processes might lead to new treatment options.

Genetic and Epigenetic Research:

- Genetic Factors: Genetic research aims to identify genetic variations associated with chronic pain susceptibility and response to treatment. By analyzing large cohorts of patients, researchers are uncovering genetic markers linked to different types of chronic pain, such as neuropathic pain or fibromyalgia. This information can guide personalized treatment approaches and improve our understanding of pain etiology.
- Epigenetic Modifications: Epigenetics refers to changes in gene expression that do not involve alterations in the DNA sequence itself. Research is exploring how epigenetic modifications, such as DNA methylation and histone modification, impact pain pathways and contribute to chronic

pain development. Understanding these mechanisms may lead to novel strategies for pain management and prevention.

2. Advances in Pharmacological Treatments

New Drug Discoveries:

- Targeted Therapies: Research is focused on developing targeted therapies that specifically modulate pain pathways or address underlying mechanisms of chronic pain. This includes the development of drugs that selectively target pain receptors or neurotransmitter systems, aiming to provide more effective pain relief with fewer side effects.

- Combination Therapies: Investigators are exploring combination therapies that involve using multiple medications or treatment modalities to enhance pain relief and reduce reliance on opioids. Studies are examining the synergistic effects of combining analgesics with anti-inflammatory agents, muscle relaxants, or antidepressants to achieve better outcomes for patients with chronic pain.

Pharmacogenomics:

- Personalized Medicine: Pharmacogenomic research is focused on understanding how genetic variations influence individual responses to pain medications. By analyzing genetic profiles, researchers aim to tailor drug treatments to individual patients, optimizing efficacy and minimizing adverse effects. This approach holds promise for personalized pain management strategies.

3. Innovations in Physical Therapy and Rehabilitation

Rehabilitation Technologies:

- Wearable Devices: Recent advancements in wearable technologies, such as smart sensors and fitness trackers, are being utilized to monitor physical activity, track movement patterns, and assess rehabilitation progress. These devices provide real-time feedback and enable personalized exercise regimens tailored to individual needs.
- Virtual Reality (VR) and Augmented Reality (AR): VR and AR technologies are being integrated into physical therapy and rehabilitation programs to create immersive environments that enhance patient engagement and motivation. These technologies offer interactive experiences for pain management, movement training, and cognitive rehabilitation.

Telehealth and Remote Monitoring:

- Telephysical Therapy: Telehealth platforms are expanding the accessibility of physical therapy by enabling remote consultations and guided exercise programs. Research is evaluating the effectiveness of telephysical therapy in managing chronic pain and comparing it to traditional in-person therapy.

- Remote Monitoring Tools: The use of remote monitoring tools, such as wearable sensors and digital health apps, is being investigated for their potential to track patient progress, adherence to exercise routines, and pain levels. These tools can provide valuable data for adjusting treatment plans and enhancing patient care.

4. Mind-Body and Integrative Approaches

Mindfulness-Based Interventions:

- Neurobiological Effects: Research is exploring the neurobiological mechanisms underlying mindfulness-based interventions, such as mindfulness-based stress reduction (MBSR) and mindfulness-based cognitive therapy (MBCT). Studies are examining how these practices influence brain function, pain perception, and emotional regulation, with the aim of improving pain management outcomes.
- Digital Mindfulness Programs: The development of digital platforms and mobile apps for mindfulness and meditation is gaining attention. Research is assessing the efficacy of these programs in managing chronic pain and enhancing overall well-being, providing patients with accessible tools for self-care.

Complementary and Alternative Therapies:

- Acupuncture and Herbal Medicine: Ongoing research is evaluating the efficacy of acupuncture and herbal medicine in managing chronic pain. Studies are investigating how these therapies may influence pain pathways, reduce inflammation, and improve quality of life for patients with chronic pain conditions.
- Biofeedback and Neurofeedback: Biofeedback and neurofeedback techniques are being explored for their potential to enhance pain management by training patients to regulate physiological responses and brain activity. Research is examining the effectiveness of these techniques in reducing pain and improving overall functioning.

5. Future Directions and Emerging Trends

Artificial Intelligence and Machine Learning:

- Predictive Analytics: AI and machine learning technologies are being applied to analyze large datasets and predict pain outcomes. Researchers are developing algorithms that can identify patterns in patient data, such as pain reports, treatment responses, and genetic information, to optimize treatment plans and improve patient outcomes.
- Personalized Treatment Models: AI-driven models are being explored to create personalized treatment recommendations based on individual

patient characteristics and preferences. These models aim to enhance decision-making and tailor interventions to each patient's unique needs.

Regenerative Medicine and Novel Therapies:

- **Stem Cell Research:** Stem cell research is investigating the potential of regenerative therapies for chronic pain management. Studies are exploring how stem cells can repair damaged tissues, modulate pain pathways, and promote healing in conditions such as osteoarthritis and neuropathic pain.
- **Gene Therapy:** Gene therapy approaches are being developed to address the underlying genetic factors contributing to chronic pain. Researchers are exploring how modifying gene expression or delivering therapeutic genes can alter pain pathways and provide long-term relief.

POTENTIAL FUTURE THERAPIES

The landscape of chronic pain management is continually evolving, driven by advancements in research and technology. Potential future therapies hold promise for transforming how chronic pain is treated, offering new avenues for relief and improving the overall quality of life for patients. This section explores some of the most exciting and innovative therapies on the horizon, focusing on their mechanisms, potential benefits, and challenges.

1. Regenerative Medicine
Stem Cell Therapy:

- Mechanism: Stem cell therapy involves using undifferentiated cells to regenerate or repair damaged tissues. In chronic pain management, stem cells are being investigated for their potential to repair injured nerves, cartilage, and other tissues that contribute to pain. Stem cells can differentiate into various cell types, potentially restoring normal tissue function and reducing pain.
- Current Research: Clinical trials are ongoing to assess the efficacy of stem cell injections for conditions such as osteoarthritis, intervertebral disc degeneration, and neuropathic pain. Researchers are exploring different types of stem cells, including mesenchymal stem cells (MSCs) and induced pluripotent stem cells (iPSCs), to determine their safety and effectiveness in pain management.
- Challenges: Despite promising early results, stem cell therapy faces challenges such as ensuring cell survival, integration into target tissues, and

long-term efficacy. Regulatory hurdles and high costs also pose obstacles to widespread adoption.

Gene Therapy:

- Mechanism: Gene therapy aims to modify or introduce genes to alter pain pathways and alleviate chronic pain. This can involve delivering therapeutic genes to produce pain-relief proteins, silencing genes that contribute to pain, or correcting genetic mutations associated with pain conditions.

- Current Research: Researchers are exploring gene therapy approaches for conditions like chronic back pain, neuropathic pain, and complex regional pain syndrome (CRPS). Techniques such as viral vector delivery and gene editing (e.g., CRISPR/Cas9) are being tested to target pain-related genes and pathways.

- Challenges: Gene therapy is still in the experimental stage, with challenges related to safe and effective delivery methods, potential immune responses, and ethical considerations. Long-term effects and sustainability of gene therapy also need further investigation.

2. Advanced Neuromodulation Techniques

Transcranial Magnetic Stimulation (TMS):

- Mechanism: TMS uses magnetic fields to stimulate specific areas of the brain involved in pain perception and modulation. By applying electromagnetic pulses, TMS aims to modulate neural activity and reduce pain.

- Current Research: Clinical trials are evaluating the effectiveness of TMS for various chronic pain conditions, including fibromyalgia, chronic migraine, and neuropathic pain. Research is focusing on optimizing treatment parameters, such as frequency and intensity, to enhance efficacy.
- Challenges: The effectiveness of TMS can vary among individuals, and research is ongoing to determine optimal treatment protocols. Long-term effects and the potential for side effects are also areas of concern.

Spinal Cord Stimulation (SCS) Innovations:

- Mechanism: SCS involves implanting a device that delivers electrical impulses to the spinal cord, modulating pain signals before they reach the brain. Innovations in SCS technology include adaptive stimulation, high-frequency stimulation, and closed-loop systems that adjust stimulation based on real-time feedback.
- Current Research: Advances in SCS technology are being explored to improve pain relief, reduce side effects, and enhance patient satisfaction. Research is focusing on optimizing stimulation parameters and exploring new device designs.

- **Challenges:** Challenges with SCS include device-related complications, such as lead migration and infection. Additionally, patient responses to SCS can vary, and long-term efficacy needs further study.

3. Personalized Medicine

Pharmacogenomics:

- **Mechanism:** Pharmacogenomics involves tailoring drug treatments based on an individual's genetic profile. By analyzing genetic variations, healthcare providers can predict how patients will respond to specific pain medications and adjust treatment accordingly.
- **Current Research:** Research is ongoing to identify genetic markers associated with pain medication efficacy and adverse effects. Personalized medicine aims to optimize drug choices and dosages, improving outcomes and minimizing side effects.
- **Challenges:** The integration of pharmacogenomics into clinical practice faces challenges such as the cost of genetic testing, the need for standardized guidelines, and ensuring accessibility for all patients.

Biomarker-Based Treatments:

- **Mechanism:** Biomarkers are biological indicators that can provide information about disease state, prognosis, or response to treatment. In chronic pain management, biomarkers can help identify specific pain mechanisms and predict treatment responses.

- Current Research: Researchers are exploring biomarkers for conditions such as osteoarthritis, rheumatoid arthritis, and neuropathic pain. The goal is to develop targeted therapies based on biomarker profiles, leading to more effective and individualized treatment approaches.
- Challenges: Identifying reliable biomarkers and validating their clinical utility can be complex. Research is needed to establish biomarker-based treatment protocols and integrate them into routine care.

4. Digital Health Innovations

Wearable Technologies:

- Mechanism: Wearable devices, such as smartwatches and fitness trackers, can monitor physiological parameters, such as activity levels, heart rate, and sleep patterns. These devices provide real-time data that can be used to manage chronic pain and assess treatment effectiveness.
- Current Research: Research is exploring the use of wearable technologies to track pain levels, medication adherence, and physical activity. Innovations in wearable devices aim to provide

personalized feedback and support self-management strategies.

- Challenges: Challenges include ensuring data accuracy, privacy concerns, and the need for user-friendly interfaces. Integration of wearable technology with existing healthcare systems also requires further development.

Telehealth and Remote Monitoring:

- Mechanism: Telehealth involves using digital platforms to provide remote consultations, therapy sessions, and monitoring. Remote monitoring tools, such as digital health apps and telehealth platforms, facilitate continuous communication between patients and healthcare providers.
- Current Research: Research is examining the effectiveness of telehealth for chronic pain management, including virtual physical therapy, remote counseling, and teleconsultations. Studies are assessing the impact of telehealth on patient outcomes, accessibility, and satisfaction.
- Challenges: Challenges include ensuring the security and privacy of patient data, addressing technological barriers, and maintaining engagement in remote care. Access to reliable internet and digital literacy are also considerations for successful implementation.

5. Integrative and Holistic Approaches

Bioelectronic Medicine:

- Mechanism: Bioelectronic medicine involves using electronic devices to modulate biological processes and treat pain. This can include neuromodulation techniques, such as bioelectronic implants and wearables, that interact with the nervous system to reduce pain.
- Current Research: Research is exploring bioelectronic devices for conditions such as chronic migraine, back pain, and neuropathic pain. Innovations aim to provide non-invasive or minimally invasive options for pain management.
- Challenges: Challenges include device safety, efficacy, and long-term outcomes. Further research is needed to understand the mechanisms of bioelectronic medicine and its potential applications.

Holistic and Integrative Therapies:

- Mechanism: Holistic approaches focus on treating the whole person, addressing physical, emotional, and spiritual aspects of health. Integrative therapies, such as yoga, tai chi, and acupuncture, are used in combination with conventional treatments to manage chronic pain.
- Current Research: Research is investigating the effectiveness of integrative therapies for various chronic pain conditions. Studies aim to understand how these therapies influence pain

perception, emotional well-being, and overall quality of life.

- Challenges: Challenges include the need for high-quality evidence supporting the efficacy of holistic therapies. Integration into conventional care requires collaboration between practitioners and consideration of patient preferences.

STAYING INFORMED AND INVOLVED

As chronic pain management continues to evolve, staying informed and actively involved in one's treatment and care is crucial for achieving the best possible outcomes. This section explores how individuals with chronic pain, caregivers, and healthcare professionals can engage with ongoing developments in the field, advocate for their needs, and participate in the broader conversation about pain management.

1. Engaging with Ongoing Research

Participating in Clinical Trials:

- Overview: Clinical trials are research studies designed to test new treatments, therapies, or interventions in a controlled environment. By participating in clinical trials, patients can access cutting-edge treatments and contribute to advancing knowledge in chronic pain management.

- How to Get Involved: Patients interested in clinical trials can search for studies through databases such as ClinicalTrials.gov or consult with their healthcare providers. They should review the eligibility criteria, potential risks, and benefits before enrolling.
- Challenges: Participation in clinical trials may involve time commitments, travel, and potential side effects. It is essential for patients to weigh these factors and discuss them with their healthcare providers before joining a trial.

Following Research Updates:

- Overview: Staying informed about the latest research findings can help individuals understand emerging treatments and advancements in chronic pain management. Research updates are often published in medical journals, presented at conferences, and discussed in professional networks.
- How to Stay Updated: Patients and caregivers can subscribe to newsletters, follow relevant medical organizations, and access online journals or research databases. Engaging with reputable sources, such as academic institutions and professional societies, ensures accurate and reliable information.
- Challenges: The volume of research can be overwhelming, and not all findings may be

relevant to every individual. It is helpful to focus on credible sources and seek guidance from healthcare providers to interpret research findings.

2. Advocating for Personal Needs

Communicating with Healthcare Providers:

- Overview: Effective communication with healthcare providers is essential for managing chronic pain. Patients should feel empowered to discuss their symptoms, treatment preferences, and concerns openly.

- How to Advocate: Patients can prepare for appointments by keeping a pain diary, listing questions or concerns, and being honest about their experiences. Building a collaborative relationship with healthcare providers can lead to more personalized and effective care.

- Challenges: Barriers to effective communication may include time constraints during appointments, language differences, or discomfort discussing certain topics. Patients should seek support from advocacy organizations or consider bringing a trusted friend or family member to appointments for additional support.

Seeking Second Opinions:

- Overview: Obtaining a second opinion can provide additional insights and treatment options, particularly for complex or challenging chronic pain cases. It offers a broader perspective on diagnosis and management strategies.

- How to Seek a Second Opinion: Patients can request referrals from their primary healthcare provider or research specialists in their condition. It is important to share relevant medical history and test results with the new provider to ensure a comprehensive evaluation.
- Challenges: Seeking a second opinion may involve additional time, cost, and effort. Patients should weigh the potential benefits and work with their healthcare team to coordinate the process.

3. Participating in Support Networks

Joining Support Groups:

- Overview: Support groups provide emotional support, practical advice, and a sense of community for individuals with chronic pain. These groups offer a space to share experiences, learn coping strategies, and connect with others facing similar challenges.
- How to Get Involved: Patients can find support groups through local hospitals, community organizations, or online platforms. Participating in both in-person and virtual groups can enhance the support network and provide diverse perspectives.

- Challenges: Finding the right support group that aligns with individual needs and preferences can be challenging. It may require trying different groups or formats to find the best fit.

Engaging in Online Forums:

- Overview: Online forums and social media platforms offer opportunities to connect with others who have chronic pain, share experiences, and access information and resources. These platforms can provide additional support and information beyond traditional settings.
- How to Engage: Patients can join online forums, follow relevant social media accounts, and participate in discussions related to chronic pain. It is important to engage with reputable and moderated forums to ensure accurate and supportive interactions.
- Challenges: Online interactions may vary in quality, and it is important to verify information from credible sources. Patients should approach online forums with a critical eye and seek professional advice when needed.

4. Staying Informed About Legal and Policy Issues

Understanding Pain Management Policies:

- Overview: Policies and regulations regarding chronic pain management can impact treatment options, access to care, and patient rights. Staying informed about these policies helps patients advocate for their needs and navigate the healthcare system effectively.

- How to Stay Informed: Patients can follow updates from regulatory agencies, professional organizations, and patient advocacy groups. Engaging with policy discussions and understanding how changes may affect pain management is essential.
- Challenges: Policy changes can be complex and difficult to follow. Patients should seek assistance from advocacy organizations or healthcare professionals to understand how policies impact their care.

Advocating for Policy Changes:

- Overview: Advocacy efforts can help shape policies and improve access to care for individuals with chronic pain. Engaging in advocacy activities, such as contacting legislators or participating in public campaigns, can drive positive change.
- How to Advocate: Patients can join advocacy organizations, participate in awareness campaigns, and communicate with policymakers about their experiences and needs. Supporting initiatives that promote research, access to care, and patient rights is crucial.
- Challenges: Advocacy efforts may require time, effort, and collaboration with others. It is

important to stay informed about ongoing initiatives and work with established organizations to maximize impact.

5. Engaging in Self-Education and Awareness

Learning About Chronic Pain Conditions:

- Overview: Educating oneself about specific chronic pain conditions and treatment options empowers individuals to make informed decisions about their care. Understanding the nature of their condition helps patients advocate for appropriate treatments and management strategies.

- How to Learn: Patients can access educational resources, attend seminars or workshops, and consult reputable medical websites. Collaborating with healthcare providers to discuss educational materials and resources is also beneficial.

- Challenges: The complexity of medical information can be overwhelming. Patients should focus on reputable sources and seek guidance from healthcare providers to ensure accurate understanding.

Promoting Awareness and Education:

- Overview: Raising awareness about chronic pain and advocating for broader education can help reduce stigma, improve public understanding, and support research efforts. Engaging in awareness campaigns and educational activities can contribute to a more informed and supportive community.

- How to Promote Awareness: Patients can participate in or organize community events, share their experiences through blogs or social media, and support organizations that focus on pain education. Collaborating with healthcare professionals and advocacy groups enhances the impact of awareness efforts.
- Challenges: Promoting awareness requires effort and engagement from multiple stakeholders. Patients should seek opportunities to collaborate with others and leverage existing platforms to maximize their reach and impact.